Third Edition

DENTAL RADIOGRAPHY:
An Introduction for Dental Hygienists and Assistants

RICHARD C. O'BRIEN, D.D.S.

Chairman
Department of Oral Radiology
Ohio State University College of Dentistry

W. B. SAUNDERS COMPANY
Philadelphia, London, Toronto

W. B. Saunders Company: West Washington Square
Philadelphia, PA 19105

1 St. Anne's Road
Eastbourne, East Sussex BN21 3UN, England

1 Goldthorne Avenue
Toronto, Ontario M8Z 5T9, Canada

Listed here is the latest translated edition of this book together
with the language of the translation and the publisher.

Spanish (*3rd Edition*) – Nueva Editorial Interamericana S.A. de C.V.,
Mexico City, Mexico

Library of Congress Cataloging in Publication Data

O'Brien, Richard C

Dental radiography.

Bibliography: p.

Includes index.

1. Teeth – Radiography.   I. Title. [DNLM;   1. Radiography, Dental. WN230 013d]

RK309.02 1977   617.6'07'572   76–8581

ISBN 0–7216–6892–5

Dental Radiography: An Introduction for Dental
Hygienists and Assistants   ISBN   0-7216-6892-5

Last digit is the print number: 9   8   7   6   5   4

PREFACE

Dental hygienists and assistants of today are highly trained to accept many more responsibilities than their counterparts of the past. One of these responsibilities is that of taking radiographs to aid in the diagnosis and treatment planning of patients. This procedure is a highly technical one and requires maximum concentration on your part because x-rays can produce harmful reactions in the human body. In order to keep to a minimum the amount of radiation delivered to a patient, a thorough knowledge of correct technique is necessary so that no radiograph will prove unacceptable because of an operator's inadequacies. It is a simple procedure, using correct technique, to re-expose the areas, but the amount of radiation absorbed when the faulty film was exposed cannot be withdrawn from the patient.

In the very near future, all persons using x-ray equipment are going to have to prove their ability and knowledge not only in technique but also in protecting the patient from excessive exposure. A number of states now require the passing of an examination before a person is permitted to operate x-ray equipment. Because this requirement is not yet universal, do not use it as an excuse for allowing yourself to become complacent. Exercise all the care and caution when exposing your patient to x-radiation that you would want another operator to use when taking an x-ray film of you!

Continual study and learning from your mistakes will enable you to become so confident that you will welcome any test to prove your ability. It is the author's wish that you will find the information in the following pages of much help in the pursuance of this objective.

RICHARD C. O'BRIEN

CONTENTS

THE NATURE AND BEHAVIOR OF X-RAYS

A man who is contented with what he has done will never become famous for what he will do.

Anonymous

Wilhelm Conrad Roentgen, along with many other scientists of his time, was experimenting with vacuum tubes. In 1895 he produced, with one of these tubes, an invisible ray that was capable of penetrating substances opaque to light. In the course of one experiment, during which the tube was covered with thick black paper, he noticed that this ray penetrated the thick paper and caused a fluorescent screen to glow. When certain objects were placed between the tube and the screen, their shadows were cast upon the screen. Further experiments proved that these rays blackened the emulsion of photographic film just as light did. Roentgen found that these rays penetrated many substances and that the shadow or image of such substances could be recorded on a photographic plate. This was true with the human body as well, and the shadows of the various body tissues — skin, muscle, and bones — could be recorded on the film. Unable to define the exact nature of this radiation, he named it the "x-ray."

ELECTROMAGNETIC RADIATIONS

It is now known that x-rays, or roentgen rays, belong to a group of electromagnetic radiations, so called because they are a combination of electric and magnetic energy. These radiations have no particles or mass but are pure energy. Corpuscular radiations, the other type of radiation, are composed of solid subatomic particles which do have mass, such as protons, electrons, neutrons, and the alpha and beta particles.

1

Radiations given off from radium and radioisotopes and during the splitting of the atom are all corpuscular in nature.

The other electromagnetic radiations are radio waves, infrared (heat) rays, ultraviolet light, gamma rays, cosmic rays, and visible light. All these rays have an undulating or wavy motion as they move through space on a straight path with a speed of 186,000 miles per second. They do differ in one respect and this is in their wave length. The wave length is the distance from the crest of one wave to the crest of the next wave (Fig. 1–1). Each radiation has its own characteristic wave length, which establishes its frequency, the frequency being the number of oscillations or waves emitted per second. Rays with shorter wave lengths therefore are of a higher frequency than those with longer wave lengths.

These radiations are arranged in the electromagnetic spectrum according to their wave lengths. Those with shorter wave lengths are measured in Angström units (one unit = 1/100,000,000 centimeter) and the longer ones are measured in meters. Each type of radiation encompasses a range of wave lengths, as can be seen in Figure 1–2. The human eye is sensitive to only a very small portion of the spectrum, that is, visible light. Color is dependent upon the wave lengths within this portion, varying from the red rays, which have the longest wave length, down to the violet rays, which have the shortest. An x-ray, with an even shorter wave length, is invisible because it is beyond the visual threshold. An important point must be emphasized here. You must always keep in mind that *x-rays are not perceptible to any of the senses*. This is what makes them so easy to ignore and why the hazards involved in their use are often overlooked.

Just as the x-rays vary in wave length, their ability to penetrate matter also varies. Those with the shorter wave length have a higher

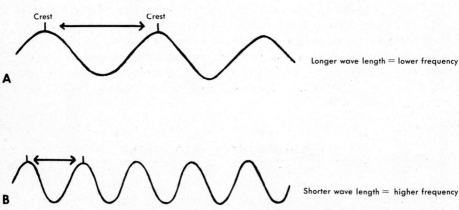

Figure 1–1   Diagram of the wave motion of an x-ray, showing measurement of the wave length. *A,* The wave length (crest to crest) is greater than that seen in *B.* Therefore it has less frequency, less energy, and therefore less ability to penetrate matter. *B,* The wave length of this ray is less than that seen in *A.* Therefore it has a higher frequency, more energy, and therefore a greater ability to penetrate matter.

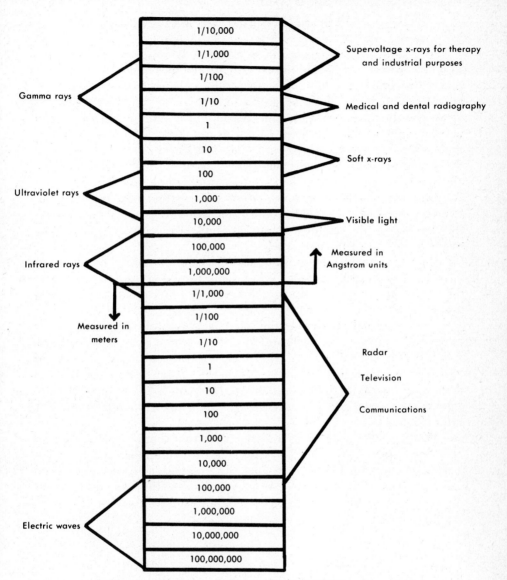

Figure 1-2 Electromagnetic spectrum.

frequency and more energy; therefore they penetrate matter with greater ease. But as the density of matter increases, the energy of the x-ray must be increased in order to penetrate it. "Hard radiation" is the term applied to the x-rays of the shorter wave lengths, and they are the ones most frequently used in medicine and dentistry. "Soft radiation" is applied to those x-rays with the longest wave lengths, and they are usually not used in dentistry because of their low energy and inability to penetrate the denser oral tissues.

PHYSICAL MAKE-UP OF MATTER

A general knowledge of the physical make-up of matter is necessary for a better understanding of x-ray production and the effects of x-rays on the body. Any form of matter, when reduced to its smallest component, is made up of atoms. For a long time it was thought that the atom was the smallest indivisible particle of an element. However, it was later found that the atom could be reduced to even smaller particles — the electrons, protons, and neutrons (Fig. 1–3).

Electrons are negative charges of electricity, protons are positive charges, and the neutrons, having no charge, are neutral. The atom has an arrangement much like a miniature solar system. The nucleus contains the positively charged protons, and when the atom has neutrons they are also in the nucleus. One or more electrons revolve around this nucleus in their respective orbits.

Because they have opposite charges, the protons and electrons have a great attraction for each other. This attraction is counteracted by the centrifugal force which maintains the position of the whirling electrons.

Under normal conditions the atom is in equilibrium; that is, it is electrically neutral. For each proton in the nucleus there is an electron in orbit. The neutron, having no charge, only adds to the atomic weight of the atom. All forms of matter are merely different arrangements of these three particles. The simplest arrangement is the hydrogen atom. The nucleus has one proton around which one electron revolves in orbit (Fig. 1–4).

If one or more electrons are removed from their respective orbits, the remainder of the atom loses its electrical neutrality and becomes positively charged. The atom is unstable in this state and is now called a positive ion. The freed electron is called a negative ion and together they are known as an ion pair. Dislodging the electron from its orbit,

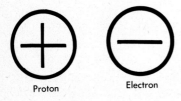

Proton   Electron   **Figure 1–3** Symbols representing a proton, an electron, and a neutron.

Neutron

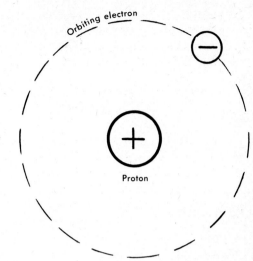

Figure 1–4 Diagrammatic representation of a hydrogen atom.

creating an ion pair, is called atom ionization (Fig. 1–5). X-rays are capable of causing this ionization of atoms to occur just as other ionizing radiations (cosmic rays, gamma rays, and corpuscular radiations) can.

Ionization of atoms of the various body tissues is therefore the basis for understanding both the therapeutic and harmful effects of x-radiation. This process can have a profound effect on the normal functional processes of a tissue when too many of its cells are altered or destroyed. Therapeutically, cancerous cells are irradiated in an attempt to destroy them before they spread. A simple example of a possible detrimental action of x-rays on the tissues is their effect on the water within

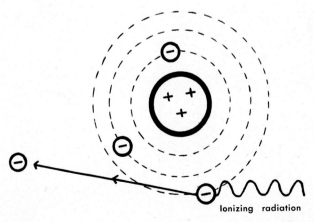

Figure 1–5 Formation of an ion pair, showing removal of an orbital electron from the energy of an x-ray.

the tissue. As the water (H_2O) absorbs the radiation energy there is a change forced on the atomic structure of the water so that it becomes hydrogen peroxide (H_2O_2). At sites where this occurs, the hydrogen peroxide, which is an oxidizing agent, causes localized tissue damage.

X-RAYS IN DENTISTRY

The study of x-radiation for diagnostic purposes is known as *radiology* or *roentgenology*. The dentist uses x-rays to record the shadows of the oral tissues on film. X-rays have the same effect on the film emulsion as ordinary light rays. The shadows of the teeth and supporting bone are projected on the film by x-rays forming a latent image which is revealed visibly once the film is processed. These films may be referred to as x-ray films, roentgenographs, roentgenograms, or radiographs.

The dental patient is subjected to both primary and secondary radiation when a dental radiograph is taken. Primary radiation is that which is emitted from the x-ray tube. Since the primary beam is used to expose the film, the patient receives mainly primary radiation. But x-rays are not reflected from an object as visible light rays are. They tend to be absorbed by the objects they strike. These objects, in turn, emit x-rays which go on to irradiate other matter in a chainlike reaction so that the entire room and the objects within it are irradiated (Fig. 1–6). All the radiation other than the primary radiation is called secondary radiation. Since it travels in all directions from an irradiated object, secondary radiation is sometimes referred to as *"scatter radiation."* It is weakened (attenuated) as it gets farther from the source of primary radiation.

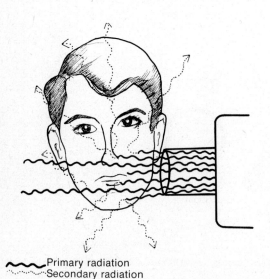

Figure 1–6 Development of secondary radiation as the primary radiation strikes the patient.

〰〰 Primary radiation
······· Secondary radiation

When we expose only a small area of tissue to the primary beam, as when we take radiographs of dental patients, the term "specific area radiation" is used. However, "whole body radiation" also occurs, since the entire body is exposed to secondary radiation.

The question is often asked, "Can I walk back into the room or close to the unit immediately after the exposure, or should I wait a few moments?" In other words, is there any lingering radiation? If you turn on a light in a dark room, the room is lighted instantly. When you turn the light off, the room becomes dark instantly. This is the exact action of x-rays. They are produced only so long as the electric current continues to generate them in the x-ray tube. When the current is turned off, x-ray production ceases instantly, the room being free of any trace of primary or secondary radiation.

HAZARDS OF RADIATION

All of us are constantly being exposed to some type of ionizing radiation. From the atmosphere there is cosmic radiation. Radiation also comes from radioactive elements in the earth and the sea. In addition to nature's radiations there are many that are man-made. Fallout, the result of atomic explosions, is an ever-increasing source, and minute amounts of radiation are emitted by such commonplace articles as the luminous dials on watches and clocks and by television sets. Medical and dental x-rays are a major source of exposure to those who are subjected to them.

It would be impossible to determine accurately the exact amount of radiation anyone receives from all sources. We do know, however, that radiation is basically harmful and that anyone who delivers radiation to another individual's tissues, as you will when exposing dental films, should be aware of the hazards involved. Irradiation of a living cell always alters the cell to some extent. The cell can be damaged slightly, temporarily interrupting its normal activity; it can be damaged permanently; or it can even die as a result of exposure. The quality and quantity of radiation delivered to the cell and the type of cell irradiated determine the end result.

Genetic and somatic cells are the two kinds of cells which make up the tissues of the human body. The genetic cells, which contain the genes, are concerned with reproduction. All other cells are classified as somatic, for example, the cells of the skin, hair, blood, glands, bone, nerves, and muscle. The different organs and body tissues respond differently to radiation. Blood-forming cells are most easily altered or destroyed by x-rays, whereas muscle and nerve cells are least likely to be affected. Within each specific organ or tissue the immature or rapidly reproducing cells are much more sensitive than the mature or dormant cells.

The injurious effects of x-radiation are cumulative. The effect of an amount of x-radiation given one time is added to that of the amount given at another time. With each dose, cellular damage is increased until there is noticeable change in the exposed tissues. This is called chronic exposure. However, with the exception of the genetic tissue, this cumulative effect depreciates over a period of time if the patient has not had further exposure. An acute overexposure occurs when a single dose of radiation causes a marked cellular change. This may be desirable, as in radiation therapy, when destruction of a tumorous growth is the result. A roentgen unit, represented by the symbol R, is the unit or measurement used to determine the amount of radiation received by a patient. The amount of cellular damage can be estimated when it is known approximately how many roentgen units were delivered to the affected tissue.

The term "latent period" is used to describe the time lapse from x-ray exposure until the damage is observable. Some reactions resulting from radiation exposure will be noticeable within a few days. Other reactions take as long as 20 years or more from the time of exposure until the effects are noticed. Those people who were exposed to radiation from the atomic bombs that fell on Japan are still suffering from the after effects. One of the results has been an increase in the incidence of leukemia.

Somatic cell injury, after the latent period, is observable in the person who was exposed to x-rays. Such injury will heal, up to a certain point. The first tissue to be irradiated during any exposure is the skin. The probable reaction from an overexposure of the skin is an erythematous reaction, a reddening of the skin similar to a sunburn. This usually appears several hours after the dose is administered. Pigmentation of the skin usually replaces the erythema a week or more after the exposure. Further exposure of the same area results in the development of scales on the skin surface, which may degenerate into persistent ulcerations. This degenerative condition is known as x-ray dermatitis and in the past developed in the fingers of many dentists who persisted in holding films in the patient's mouth during exposure. Before the dangers of radiation were fully realized this occurred quite frequently. Loss of hair, either temporary or permanent, can also occur following excessive exposure to x-rays. The chances of this happening as a result of conventional intraoral roentgenographic examination are highly remote. The cells of the lens of the eye are incapable of reproducing themselves; therefore, caution should be exercised to avoid exposing the eye to any unnecessary radiation. For added protection the patient can be instructed to close his eyes during exposure. Although there are reactions from overexposure in other structures of the body, such as the blood-forming organs or glandular tissue, erythema is the most likely reaction to be experienced as a result of exposure to an excessive amount of dental x-rays.

An injurious amount of x-radiation to the reproductive organs may cause genetic cell injury involving a mutation of the chromosomes in the patient's ova or sperm. The damage to the chromosomes is permanent, although not all the chromosomes may be involved. If a sperm or ovum carrying a mutated chromosome is involved in fertilization, the damage may be observable in the patient's offspring or in future generations, depending upon the type and severity of the mutation. Such mutations passed from one generation to another may be further changed by additional radiation, and these accumulated mutations are passed on to future offspring. The reproductive cells of the male, located in the testes, are much more vulnerable to radiation than those of the female, which are protected by the deep internal location of the ovaries. The reproductive cells of the female patient receive less than half as much radiation from oral x-rays as do those of the male. However, when taking radiographs of a pregnant woman, you must keep in mind that the fetus she carries is a mass of rapidly multiplying cells, especially in the first trimester. This patient must be given every possible protection, including a lead apron to cover the abdomen.

Precautions

In spite of these hazards, routine dental radiography is well within the safe limits of exposure if proper precautions are taken. Correct adjustment of the x-ray equipment insures that the size of the x-ray beam is just enough to permit a minimum of area exposure within practical limits. Proper filtration of the primary beam eliminates the less penetrating rays, which are of no value since they do not act on the film but are merely absorbed by the patient. Use of the fastest film possible requires less exposure time per film. The patient should be questioned about any previous exposure, such as medical x-rays, x-ray treatment, and dental x-rays, and, if known, about the radiation dose received in each instance. It should also be noted how long it has been since the last exposure, for the cumulative effects diminish over a period of time.

The dentist must evaluate this information and make the final decision whether the x-rays should be taken. However, only in the most unusual circumstances will he decide that a patient should not have a routine dental radiographic examination because of previous radiation. There is little danger of cumulative damage from taking dental radiographs, since there is normally an interval of 6 months or longer between exposures. Responsible personnel in the dental office should be satisfied with nothing less than perfection in their radiographic technique. This will eliminate any need for retakes of intraoral and extraoral radiographs, making further exposure unnecessary.

THE RELUCTANT PATIENT

If a patient hesitates or totally rejects the idea of being exposed to x-rays, there is a tendency among some dentists to discontinue treatment. The dentist does not wish to perform his services on someone who allows only a partial diagnosis of his condition. Because he is responsible for his patient's welfare, he cannot be reproached for this decision. However, with a minimum of effort many of these patients can be persuaded to accept dental radiography. These are the people who become missionaries for the dentist and his practice because time has been taken to explain the nature and facts of a subject that is of concern to the patient.

Quite often the source of a patient's misgivings about x-rays is something he has read. Most articles and items are based on fact; however, closer examination of some of them may reveal that they were based on erroneous information, misquotations, and misinterpretations. They are convincing because they were published and also because the author was enthusiastically convincing in writing what he believed to be true. Laymen who alert the public to the dangers of x-radiation prove the old saying that a little knowledge is a dangerous thing.

There are other reasons for reluctance to be x-rayed; chief among them are financial reasons, failure to comprehend the necessity for radiographs, and an innate fear of the unfamiliar. But we have at our disposal the means by which we can convince misinformed, reluctant patients of the need for radiographs. We have access to the latest information on x-radiation and, more importantly, the ability to understand it and apply it. Our motivation to favorably influence these patients is the knowledge that without radiographs we cannot properly treat them.

Motivate Yourself First

The prerequisite to patient education is self-education. Make every effort to obtain the latest information about x-radiation, for the better informed you are, the more able you will be to present the most up-to-date facts. It is mainly through patient education that the true facts are made known to the public.

To convince patients of the necessity of taking radiographs, be convinced of that necessity yourself. Then your own enthusiasm for the values and benefits he will receive by the use of x-rays will transmit itself to him. However, unless you can demonstrate these advantages, a patient may remain uncooperative in spite of your enthusiasm.

Proper presentation of these facts is a primary concern. Present them in an orderly manner so they can be considered carefully. Beyond any doubt, make sure that what you say is accurately understood by your patient. Though you are informed on the subject, very few laymen have any real degree of understanding of x-rays. Therefore, keep your discussions as elementary as possible, leaving no "blank spots" in the presentation. Keep in mind that people are not impressed by what you say but rather by what they understand. Too often an attempt to impress patients only confuses them. Confused thoughts will rapidly close an open mind.

Keeping the Upper Hand

The disturbing effect of unfavorable articles is that the dentist or hygienist is placed on the defensive. This renders the efforts of educating patients to accept oral radiographic procedures all the more trying. When presenting our side of the story, don't be misled by assuming that the door to the patient's mind is wide open and all you must do is speak and the patient will accept your word as being infallible. He is under the influence of too many external factors which have helped him arrive at his own conclusions.

When x-rays are the topic of discussion, the patient must be willing to listen to what you have to say. He must open his mind to the facts you present, just as he did to those who caused him to have this fear in the first place. He must be in a receptive mood. You can usually assume there is an interest in what you are saying if questions are asked with the purpose in mind of gaining more information. If, on the other hand, a patient makes definite statements in opposition to your explanation to him, you may as well save your efforts until he is in a more receptive mood. He is not interested in what you have to say but merely in asserting his own opinion.

Some Pertinent Facts

Every human being is constantly exposed to radiation from outer space and from the earth. This is known as *background radiation*. According to the National Research Council of the National Academy of Sciences, "the average exposure of the population's reproductive cells to radiation above the natural background should be limited to 10 roentgen (R) from conception to age 30." You, as a user of x-rays, are permitted a higher safety dose. Any minor mutations that may take place within you as a result of your continuous daily exposure will be absorbed by the general population.

However, your patient is not concerned with the general public but rather with what is taking place within him. When x-raying the patient's oral tissues, a minute amount of this radiation registers its effect on the reproductive cells via secondary radiation. Richards found this to be approximately 1/10,000 of the amount of specific-area radiation delivered to the oral tissues. With female patients there would be only one-fifth to one-seventh of this amount because of the internal location of their reproductive organs. With a properly controlled unit and with the most sensitive film possible, a routine full-mouth examination would expose the patient to approximately 5 to 6 R (65 KVP, 10 MA). This would be specific-area radiation delivered to the face, of which approximately .0005 R of x-radiation would reach the reproductive cells of the male. It is estimated that everyone receives approximately .0004 R per day to the reproductive cells from background radiation. By comparing these figures we see that a patient's reproductive tissues receive radiation from a full-mouth examination in amounts slightly higher than that which he receives from daily background radiation.

Because patients seem to understand dental x-ray dosage better when compared to other areas of radiation, you might wish to provide them with a few of these comparisons, such as the following (all refer to genetic exposure):

He would receive approximately 1 mR from a chest film.
He would receive approximately 1000 mR from a gastrointestinal series.
If he were to reside in a masonry or brick house over a 30-year period, he would receive approximately 1300 mR from the building materials.
Persons living in areas of high elevation will receive in a 30-year period 500 mR more than those living at sea level.

A Probable Source of Our Problem

It is interesting to note how some of the information which caused the uproar over injurious effects of dental x-rays originated. An article in J.A.D.A. by William E. Nolan (1953) proved enlightening. It is well written, and at the time, it presented to the profession much revealing data. However, many quotations were dispensed through the various news media to the general public. The facts thus presented may have been accurate, but they were often misinterpreted, misquoted, and exaggerated.

First of all, these misconceptions are based on an article written 24 years ago. It shouldn't be too difficult to impress a patient with the fact that such information can't be applied to the newer radiographic techniques and equipment.

Specifically, Nolan stated that one patient received 315 R during a full-mouth examination. Several other patients received between 280 and 300 R. In light of today's knowledge these are rather frightening figures. Once this information reached the radio and newspapers, we couldn't blame the general public for giving dental x-rays a second thought.

It may seem incredible that a patient could receive such quantities of x-radiation during a full-mouth examination. However, if you were to read this article you would find the following reasons:

1. The units used to make up these data had no filtration and were poorly collimated.
2. The number of exposures used to complete the full-mouth examination varied from 25 to 35.
3. The films used were the slower speed type.

In comparing present-day x-ray procedures with the above, we see the following:

1. The modern units of today are accurately filtered to eliminate most of the useless x-rays and are properly collimated.
2. The number of films used in a full-mouth examination rarely exceeds 20 and is usually less.
3. The outstanding factor in the reduction of x-rays delivered to the patient is the development of high-speed films.

Another highly significant fact is that Nolan states that the x-rays were delivered "to the region." In dentistry, x-rays are delivered to a small, specific area. Most patients do not understand this and relate any dosage delivered to the region of the face and neck as being whole body radiation. When they hear from the news media that "so many" radiation units can cause bodily injury, it is not fully explained that this pertains to radiation delivered to the whole body. This is not so for patients receiving dental x-rays and should be clarified.

When considering the total amount of radiation units a patient receives from specific-area radiation, it is sometimes referred to as being collectively received at a certain point, such as the tongue or thyroid. Though the general area of the face and neck receives the brunt of the x-rays, it is doubtful that there is a certain point where all the rays intersect. Therefore, no well-defined area receives the total accumulative amount of administered radiation.

Through the years from 1953 to the present, we have seen definite improvements in our x-ray procedures, to a point where our patients may receive only 5 to 6 R per full-mouth examination. We can attribute most of this reduction to the development of highly sensitive films, although proper filtration and smaller beam collimators have also contributed. With this in mind it is all but impossible to give the patient enough radiation (250 R) to cause an erythema that would be visible and alarming.

Your Patient's Fears

Actually there are only two areas in which the patient usually expresses concern: change in the blood and lymphatic tissues and genetic alteration. The genetic changes generally concern those patients under 40, since most children are conceived at this time. It is usually not a factor beyond this age. There is no known threshold dose above which there is genetic damage or below which there is none. Regardless of how small the dose, it has an accumulative effect which, with subsequent x-rays, could build to a point at which it could be observed in some future offspring. It is generally agreed that no adverse effects will be encountered, either by the patient or his offspring, if the National Academy of Science's 10-R recommendation is not exceeded. However, it is your moral obligation to keep the amount of radiation you deliver to the patient at the lowest possible level, since dental radiographs are a fraction of the total 10-R limitation.

As far as blood cell changes are concerned, Nolan stated that there were noticeable changes in the patients he observed for his article. Considering the large amounts of radiation they received, this is not surprising, but it is highly unlikely that in your patients a routine dental radiographic examination will adversely affect the blood-forming tissues or blood cells if you follow all safety recommendations.

A Case In Point

One of my patients, who was opposed to having a series of x-rays taken, had evidently been reading quite a bit about the dangers of such a procedure. Upon questioning her I discovered that she had read that the 15 to 20 radiographs needed to complete a full-mouth radiographic examination were exposed with x-rays directed toward the pelvic and reproductive organs. We know that there are usually only three (at most, five) exposures in which the x-rays are directed toward a point anywhere near the pelvic region, and this is with the bisecting-angle technique. When using the paralleling technique with an extended cone, all exposures are taken with the x-rays directed perpendicular to the long axis of the teeth, maintaining a still safer path for the x-rays to travel. This patient also explained that some x-ray units delivered as much as 325 R at a single setting (most likely from an article relating to Nolan's findings) and the imminent dangers to a patient absorbing so much radiation at one time. As previously noted, these dangers were associated with whole body radiation, and the large dosage of radiation was due to the use of outdated units and slow film.*

This case history is probably very similar to ones with which you are confronted. However, with Richards' findings at your disposal you have the facts with which to help the patient correct his erroneous thinking.

"Are X-rays Really Necessary?"

What will you say if your patient asks, "Why are you taking these x-rays?" A knowledgeable, simple answer by you can dispel any apprehen-

---

*R. C. O'Brien, D.D.S.

sion and build a high professional stature for you. Some of you reading this book may be experienced at answering these questions, but for those who are not the following dialogue might be helpful.

Patient: Do you have to take these x-rays?

You: Yes, the doctor has requested them.

Patient: Can't he look into my mouth and see what needs to be done?

You: More than 50 per cent of the decayed areas in teeth are discovered only through x-ray findings. Those cavities that form between the teeth, especially the bicuspids and molars, can't be seen by an oral examination. That is, of course, if the decayed area hasn't grown so large that the enamel has been undermined and broken down. In that case the hole in the tooth is quite obvious. We want to restore the tooth long before this happens.

Patient: I didn't realize that he couldn't find all the cavities with the mirror and other instruments. But why do you take so many? Wouldn't just a few x-rays show all the decay that he couldn't find otherwise?

You: The doctor has to see not only how the teeth look but how the supporting bone of your teeth looks as well. Many times the gums cover up infection that is slowly destroying this bone. Only a series of x-rays which include all areas of the mouth will show this infection if it's present.

Patient: I have been having trouble with my gums lately. They bleed slightly when I brush my teeth so I'll be very interested in what the doctor finds.

You: I don't see all your third molars. Have you had any of them removed? Impacted third molars have caused many problems which we would like to prevent from happening to you. An x-ray will readily reveal any impactions.

Patient: I believe I have had a third molar extracted. Are there any other reasons for taking an x-ray of my teeth?

You: Yes, though we don't expect to find anything seriously wrong in your mouth, the x-ray picture might reveal a bone-destroying cyst or an abscess. Most of the time there are no symptoms in the early stages of cyst and abscess development so patients aren't aware that these lesions are present. Therefore, an x-ray will show such lesions when they are more easily treated.

Patient: I can understand now why the doctor needs these x-rays and I appreciate your taking time to answer my questions.

You: The doctor will examine your mouth now, check your x-rays, and explain his findings to you.

There are certain patients for whom the preceding answers will not suffice. These are children and edentulous patients. When a mother brings her child in for an x-ray examination, these points should be made clear: (1) x-rays are necessary to detect interproximal decaying areas so that the primary teeth can be saved for function and for space maintenance for the erupting permanent teeth; and (2) only x-rays enable the doctor to observe the presence and growth process of the permanent teeth. A problem revealed by the x-ray in this area can be intercepted and dealt with.

If the patient is edentulous (no teeth present in the mouth), he may be skeptical as to why the x-ray procedure is necessary for him. Only the innocent-looking gums are seen when looking in the mouth. They may cover up root tips which are foci for infection, cysts in the bone, or impacted teeth lodged in the denture-supporting ridges—all of which can only be discovered by x-ray. When it is necessary for the doctor to remove excess tissue to provide a more stable ridge for the denture, the x-ray picture will reveal the amount of tissue to be removed.

For Your Safety

We have seen that the chances of overexposing the patient usually are remote, but how about you? You are in the operatory taking x-rays day after day over a prolonged period of time. But if you take two simple precautions when operating the x-ray unit you too will remain well within the safe limits. The first precaution is that you should never hold a film in the patient's mouth during an exposure, regardless of the circumstances, as this would put your fingers and hand in the path of the intense primary beam. The second precaution is to stand behind a protective barrier, such as a lead shield or a protective wall, during the actual exposure time. If this is not possible, stand at least 6 feet from the x-ray unit and never in the direct line of the primary beam. The activating button of the unit is on the end of a coiled extension cord, which enables you to move to one of these positions.

You must always be alert to the fact that secondary radiation can be just as harmful to you as primary radiation. It is this form of radiation that you will be exposed to most. In the dental operatory the three major sources of secondary radiation are the filter in the tube head (Fig. 2–4), the soft tissues of the patient's face, and the pointed plastic cone. All three give off this radiation simultaneously during the exposure time (Fig. 1–7). The first two sources cannot be eliminated, and the greater the distance you place between yourself and these secondary sources, the better. If you are 6 feet from the patient you will be exposed to approximately one quarter of the amount of secondary radiation you would receive at 3 feet.

Something can be done, however, about the cone. You will notice in the upcoming chapters that some of the drawings and photographs illustrate a tube head with a pointed plastic cone, while others illustrate the tube head with a rounded open-end cone. Because both types

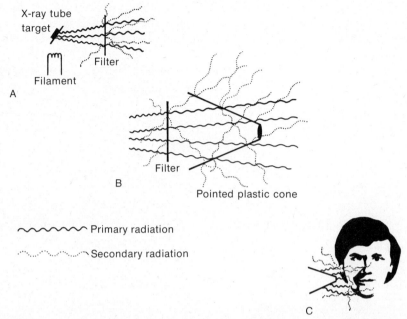

X-ray tube target

Filter

Filament

A

Filter

B

Pointed plastic cone

Primary radiation

Secondary radiation

C

Figure 1–7 Diagrammatic sketch illustrating the three major sources of secondary radiation. *A,* Primary x-rays from the x-ray tube target strike the aluminum filter, which in turn produces secondary radiation. *B,* Primary x-rays passing through the filter strike the pointed plastic cone, which in turn produces secondary radiation. *C,* Primary x-rays emerge from pointed plastic cone to strike the patient, who in turn produces secondary radiation.

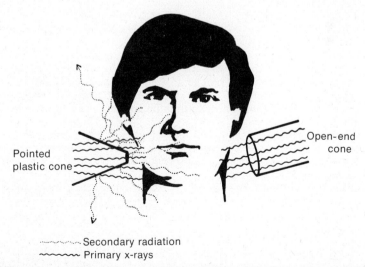

Open-end cone

Pointed plastic cone

Secondary radiation

Primary x-rays

Figure 1–8 Pointed plastic cone acts as a major source of secondary radiation when irradiated by primary radiation. This source of secondary radiation is eliminated when the open-end cone is used.

of cones are currently in use, both have been illustrated, but the pointed cones *should not be used.* All up-to-date dental x-ray units are equipped with lead-lined open-end cones. You can compare the difference in the amount of secondary radiation emitted from the cones in Figure 1–8.

There are many excellent books written about x-rays in dentistry. Some are listed below for the student who wishes to go into greater detail.

REFERENCES

Ennis, L. M., Berry, H. M., and Phillips, J. E.: Dental Roentgenology. 6th ed. Philadelphia, Lea & Febiger, 1967.

Langland, O. E., and Sippy, F. H.: Textbook of Dental Radiography. Springfield, Ill., Charles C Thomas, 1973.

Nolan, W. E.: Radiation hazards to the patient from oral roentgenology. J.A.D.A. 47:681, 1953.

Richards, A. G., et al.: X-ray protection in the dental office. J.A.D.A. 56:514, 1958.

Richards, A. G.: New method for reduction of gonadal irradiation of dental patients. J.A.D.A. 65:1, 1962.

Stafne, E. C., and Gibilisco, J. A.: Oral Roentgenographic Diagnosis. 4th ed. Philadelphia, W. B. Saunders Co., 1975.

Wainwright, W. W.: Dental Radiology. New York, McGraw-Hill Book Co., 1965.

Wuehrmann, A. H., and Manson-Hing, L. R.: Dental Radiology. 3rd ed. St. Louis, C. V. Mosby Co., 1973.

REMINDERS

1. X-rays are pure energy having no mass or particles.
2. X-rays, like light waves, travel in wavelike motion at the speed of 186,000 miles per second.
3. X-rays of shorter wave length have more energy and penetrate matter with greater ease than those with longer wave lengths.
4. When a stable atom has one of its electrons displaced from its orbit, the atom has become electrically unstable or ionized. An x-ray has the ability to ionize atoms and can thus be spoken of as "ionizing radiation."
5. Ionization of atoms making up molecules of living tissue is the basic cause of alteration of the normal chemical make-up of the tissue.
6. The patient receives both primary and secondary radiation during exposure to dental x-rays.
7. There is no lingering radiation in the operatory following patient exposure.
8. Cells making up living tissue may be spoken of as genetic (reproductive) and somatic (general).
9. Injurious effects of x-radiation are cumulative.
10. Overexposure to x-radiation is of two types—acute and chronic.
11. Injury to the somatic cells is observable in the person being radiographed. Injury to chromosomes (reproductive cells) may be manifest in future offspring.

2

THE EQUIPMENT — UNIT,
FILM, DARK ROOM

Many men and women fail in life, not for lack
of ability, or brains, or even courage, but
simply because they have never organized
their energies around a central goal.

Elmer Wheeler

THE X-RAY UNIT

Before learning the techniques of taking x-rays it is necessary to become familiar with the x-ray machine. The machine is composed of three parts: the tube head, from which the x-rays are generated; the control panel, which contains the regulating devices; and the arm, which enables you to position the tube head (Fig. 2–1).

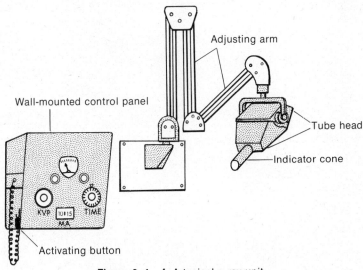

Figure 2–1 *A,* A typical x-ray unit.

Illustration continues on the following page.

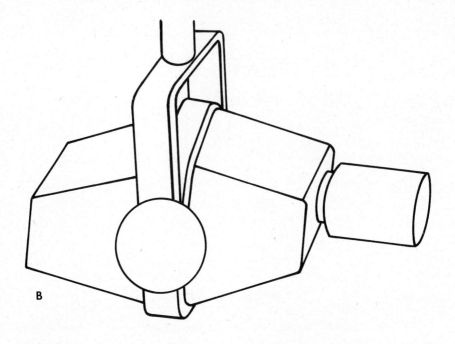

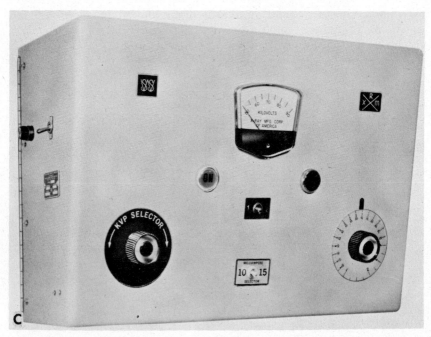

Figure 2–1 *(Continued).* B, The tube head which houses the x-ray tube. C, Timer and control panel with a range of 50 to 90 kv., with 10 and 15 ma. variable control unit.

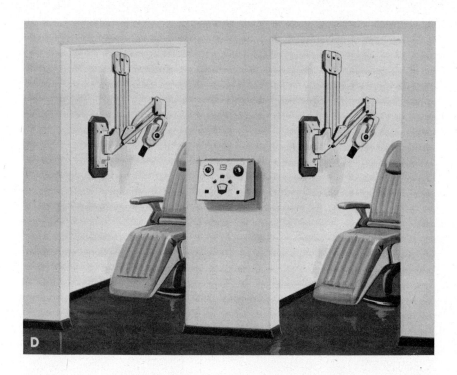

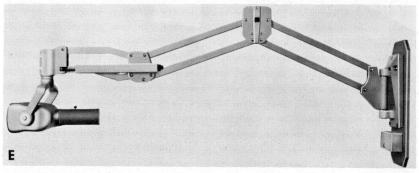

Figure 2-1 *(Continued).* *D,* Many dental offices now have a central control panel that operates two or more x-ray units. *E,* The tube head is attached to a flexible extension arm which allows it to be moved to different positions. (*C* to *E* courtesy of the S. S. White Dental Mfg. Co., X. R. M. Division.)

The tube head holds the x-ray tube; this tube is the most important component of the entire unit because it is within the tube that the x-rays are produced. Basically the tube is composed of three main parts. They are the glass envelope, the target (anode), and the filament (cathode) (Fig. 2-2).

The glass envelope houses the other two parts and is similar to the glass envelope of an ordinary light bulb. However, this envelope has lead incorporated into the glass except in that portion of the tube from

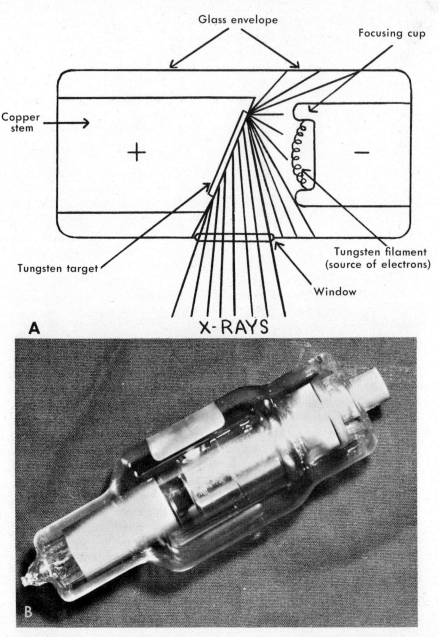

Figure 2-2 *A*, Diagrammatic sketch of an x-ray tube. *B*, Photograph of an actual x-ray tube. (*B* courtesy of the General Electric Co.)

which the primary beam makes its exit. This area, made of ordinary glass, is called the window. The purpose of the lead glass is to inhibit the passage of those x-rays not used in the primary beam through the glass envelope.

The target, or anode, is rectangular in shape and composed of tungsten. It is imbedded in a copper stem at one end of the tube. At the other end of the tube is a tungsten filament or coil (cathode) imbedded in a molybdenum focusing cup. When the activating button is pressed, the preheating stage of the tube is initiated.

During this stage the tungsten coil is heated until it glows by a low voltage current of electricity (Fig. 2–3). This glowing effect, or incandescence, is an electron cloud similar to that seen in the burning filament of a tungsten light bulb. Heating causes metals to give up some of their electrons, and a tungsten coil is used in this case because it is an excellent source of electrons. Once the desired quantity of electrons is produced by preheating the filament, a high voltage charge of electricity, which comes from a separate high voltage line, propels the electrons toward the target with tremendous speed. These electrons encounter no interference from air molecules because the tube has been evacuated of air. The focusing cup, which houses the filament, focuses the freed electrons on an area of the target known as the focal spot. When the electrons strike this focal spot, two reactions occur; heat and radiant energy are produced. This characteristic energy, which can be produced only in this manner, is known as x-radiation.

The production of x-rays works on the ionization principle described in Chapter 1. The electrons traveling at high speed from the tungsten coil strike the orbital electrons of atoms making up the tungsten target. When a high speed electron is suddenly stopped by colliding with another electron it gives up its energy in the form of high energy (short wave length) x-radiation. A partial or glancing collision will result in the electron giving up only a portion of its energy in the form of a lower energy (longer wave length) x-ray as it continues on a diverted path. Additional x-rays are produced when a target electron is dislodged from its respective orbit. As the unstable atom attracts a free electron to restore its equilibrium the process releases energy in the form of x-rays.

The heat produced within the target of the tube during the generation of the x-rays should be dissipated as soon as possible. Although

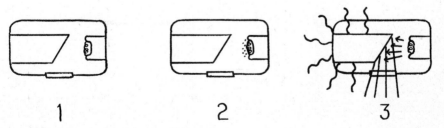

Figure 2–3 Action of the x-ray tube. *1.* Press activating button. *2.* Electron cloud formation (MA). *3.* Propulsion of electrons to target (KVP).

tungsten has a very high melting point, overheating could cause melting or pitting of the target. Tungsten is a poor heat conductor, but copper is an excellent one; therefore the target is imbedded in a copper stem. This stem rapidly conducts the heat away from the target. The heat is then absorbed, in some units, by a specially refined oil in which the tube is immersed. Other units liberate the heat to a special gas through a system of fins incorporated into the copper stem.

There are two transformers housed in the tube head unit along with the x-ray tube (Fig. 2–4). A transformer regulates voltage and is necessary because the line voltage coming to most dental offices is 220 volts, but the x-ray tube operates on both higher and lower voltages than this. Therefore the low voltage transformer is needed to produce a

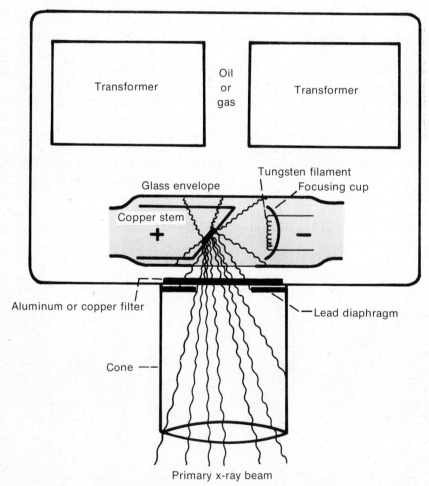

Figure 2–4 Schematic drawing of the tube head.

current of 3 to 5 volts which heats the tungsten coil. The high voltage transformer produces a voltage of 55,000 to 90,000 volts which propels the electrons.

The control panel has the devices for regulating the x-ray beam, the on-off switch, and the activating button which is at the end of a coiled extension cord. The regulating devices are the kilovoltage peak regulator (KVP), the milliamperage regulator (MA), and the timer. The dentist is responsible for determining the settings on the dials, but auxiliary personnel must understand their functions.

The kilovoltage peak control regulates the high voltage current, which in turn regulates the speed of the electrons traveling from the tungsten coil to the target. The higher the kilovoltage peak, the faster the electrons will travel. An electron with greater force (high KVP) is needed to dislodge the target electrons which occupy the orbits closest to the nucleus. Those electrons occupying the innermost orbits have a greater attraction to the nucleus than those in the outer orbits. When the target electron from one of the inner orbits is dislodged, the capture of a free electron by the unstable atom produces a harder, more energetic x-ray than that produced when one of the outer orbital electrons is dislodged (Fig. 2–5). Since a greater force is needed to dislodge one of the inner orbital electrons, the higher KVP produces x-rays with shorter wave lengths by increasing the speed of the electrons to the target. Although increased voltage produces x-rays having a shorter wave length, all the x-rays at a particular moment are heterogeneous (have many dif-

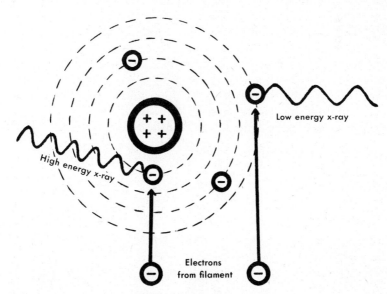

Low energy x-ray

High energy x-ray

Electrons
from filament

Figure 2–5 Diagrammatic sketch of a target atom being bombarded by electrons from the filament.

ferent wave lengths) because many electrons from all orbits of the target atoms are dislodged. The KVP is regulated to provide an x-ray beam that will penetrate to the degree desired by the dentist.

The milliamperage regulator determines the quantity of x-rays produced during the exposure by controlling the temperature of the tungsten coil. The higher the MA, the hotter the tungsten coil will become and the greater will be the number of electrons produced in the electron cloud to be propelled to the target.

The timer regulates the length of time the current will pass through the x-ray tube. The length of time needed to adequately expose the film varies greatly from 1/20 second or less to 3 or 4 seconds. In the various film packages the manufacturer includes recommended time exposures for each technique in which the film is used. These exposures are determined by the distance from the target of the x-ray tube to the film, film speed, KVP and MA, and the density of the tissues being examined. The total quantity of x-rays produced is often expressed as milliampere seconds (MAS), a milliampere second being the product of the MA and the exposure time in seconds. The greater the MAS, the more x-rays produced.

Two devices that reduce the total x-ray exposure the patient receives are incorporated in the tube head. The first of these is a filter placed in the path of the primary beam before it exits from the unit (Fig. 2–4). Only those x-rays with shorter wave lengths pass through the tissues to expose the film; therefore the less penetrating x-rays serve no useful purpose and act only to further radiate the patient. The filters, usually copper or aluminum disks, are 1/4 millimeter in thickness. They absorb most of these longer wave length rays so that the patient receives, for the most part, only those rays which are capable of exposing the film (Fig. 2–6). These filters are built into modern x-ray units by the manufacturer, but more filtration can be added by the dentist if he wishes. As the x-ray beam passes from the tube some of the weaker x-rays are absorbed by the glass tube, the oil in which the tube is immersed, and the cone tip (except the open end cones). The amount of filtration afforded by these materials is usually spoken of as being equivalent to a specific amount of aluminum and is termed "inherent

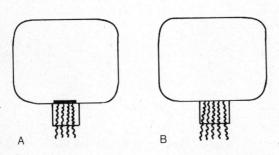

Figure 2–6 *A,* X-ray beam with proper filtration. *B,* Without filtration.

A   B

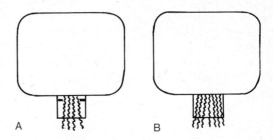

Figure 2–7 *A,* X-ray beam with collimation. *B,* Without collimation.

A   B

filtration." The increase of the filtration by the addition of the copper or aluminum disks is known as "added filtration." This added filtration plus the inherent filtration equals the "total filtration" of the unit.

The second device is a diaphragm which collimates or adjusts the size of the x-ray beam (Fig. 2–4). The diaphragm is a lead disk located at the junction of the tube head and the cone. In the center of the disk is an opening through which the x-rays pass; these x-rays comprise the useful beam, the x-rays in the center being termed the central rays (CR). The size of the useful beam is no more than 2½ to 3 inches in diameter at the tip of the cone. The smaller the opening in the diaphragm, the smaller the useful beam (Fig. 2–7). A smaller beam necessitates more accuracy when directing it toward the film during exposure. The peripheral rays are absorbed by the lead disk itself.

As the x-ray beam passes through the diaphragm it assumes the shape of a cone. The intensity of the beam is the greatest at the point of emergence, but as the beam progresses from the diaphragm the rays spread over an ever-increasing circle, becoming less and less intense. Intensity is an important consideration when adjusting the controls of the unit for the various techniques.

There are newer x-ray units now capable of taking panoramic radiographs of both maxillary and mandibular arches with one exposure. A radiograph of this type is most useful in orthodontics, periodontics, and surgery. The panoramic film is exposed extraorally; therefore some detail is lost when compared to intraoral radiographs. However, this is not objectionable when you take into consideration the amount of information that is provided.

THE FILM

The film itself has a firm but flexible polyester base. It adapts easily as it is transported smoothly through the rollers in the new automatic processors. Also, this film base does not absorb water; therefore it dries rapidly in the drying chamber. An emulsion of silver halide crystals mixed with gelatin is spread in an extremely thin layer over both sides of the base. Films for film holders and cassettes are packaged in a box, with each film individually wrapped in a black paper envelope. A film packet is made to be placed in the mouth; therefore it has an outer wrapping of paper to protect the film from moisture and light. One side of the wrapping is stippled; this helps prevent slipping when the film is positioned in the mouth. This stippled side is always placed on the tube side—that is, on the side facing the x-rays. Within the packet on the other side of the film is a lead foil backing, its purpose being to absorb as much exit radiation passing through the film as possible. It also helps to prevent fogging (darkening of the film) caused by secondary radiation created in the tissues behind the film. Immediately surrounding the film itself is a black paper envelope.

Single film packets are used if only one copy of the x-ray is desired. A double film packet containing two separate films can be used if duplicate copies of the radiograph are needed.

The speed of the film denotes the rapidity with which the film becomes adequately exposed. Basically the speeds are slow, medium, and fast or "high" speed. All other factors remaining constant, the slow speed film requires the longest exposure time, whereas fast film requires the shortest time and therefore exposes the patient to the least amount of radiation.

There are three basic types of intraoral films; each is named according to the radiographic technique with which it is used. The most frequently used is the periapical film. As the name implies, the root apex of the tooth and the surrounding structures are of prime interest when this type of film is used. There are three sizes of periapical films. No. 0 is $7/8$ by $1^3/8$ inches, for use with children. No. 1 is $^{15}/_{16}$ by $1^9/_{16}$ inches, for use in the anterior region of adult mouths when a narrow film is recommended. No. 2, the standard size, is $1^1/4$ by $1^5/8$ inches and is designed for routine use in all areas of adult mouths (Fig. 2–8).

Another exposure quite frequently taken is the bite-wing. This exposure is used mainly to detect interproximal decay and also to determine the height of the alveolar crest of the bone which supports the

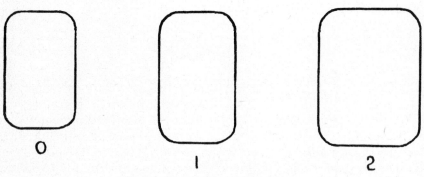

Figure 2–8   Periapical film sizes.

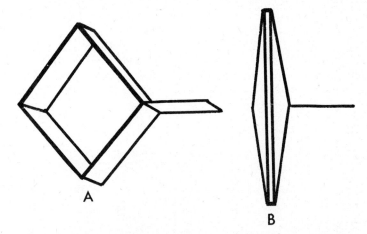

Figure 2–9 *A,* Bite-wing tab. *B,* Tab with periapical film in place.

teeth. The film has a bite-wing tab attached to it which divides the film in half through its long axis; the same film used for periapical exposures can be placed in a bite-wing tab (Fig. 2–9). The bite-wing film is put in place in the patient's mouth so that its upper half is adjacent to the maxillary teeth and its lower half adjacent to the mandibular teeth when the patient bites on the tab.

There are four sizes of bite-wing films. The extra long or No. 3 size is 1¹/₁₆ by 2¹/₈ inches. Only one No. 3 bite-wing for each side is needed for radiographs of the molars and bicuspids. The standard No. 2 size periapical film can be used for molar bite-wing exposures, but in this case a separate bicuspid film is also needed. For radiographs of the anterior teeth in adult patients a No. 1 or No. 2 size bite-wing is used. A No. 0 is used for all bite-wings in small children.

To expose larger areas of the dental arch on a single film, the occlusal film is used. On this film we can view a cross section of the teeth and the complete palatal structure. This technique is employed for determining the location of cystic lesions, impacted teeth, salivary duct stones, bone fractures, or for any reason in which the area of interest is larger than the area of the periapical size film. The occlusal film is 2¹/₄ by 3 inches and it may be used intraorally or extraorally, depending upon the situation.

Extraoral film, as the term implies, is always placed outside the patient's mouth. These films are needed for large areas of pathological involvement, impacted teeth, temporomandibular joint exposures, head plates, fractures of facial bones, and for patients who cannot open their mouths for intraoral film placement. These films are much larger than intraoral films, ranging in size from 5 by 7 inches up to 10 by 12 inches or more.

If you are going to radiograph either side of the mandible, as in the case of a lateral jaw exposure, the film should be placed in a cardboard film holder. Other extraoral exposures, such as the temporomandibular joint, require the use of a cassette to hold the film. Either a film holder or a cassette is necessary to keep the film rigid during the exposure. If the film is not kept flat the resultant image will be distorted.

A film holder (exposure holder) is two pieces of cardboard hinged

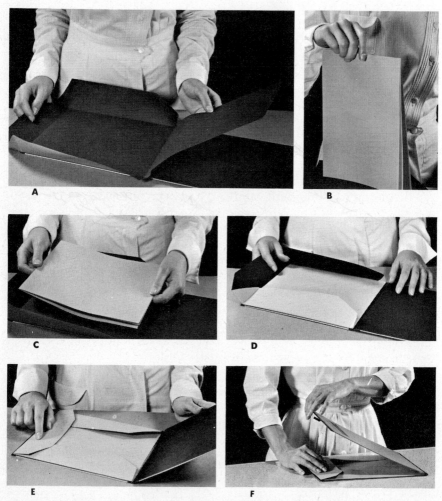

Figure 2–10 Loading exposure holder: *A,* Unlatch clip of exposure holder; raise back of holder and open paper envelope. *B,* Remove film in its protective paper folder from box with right hand and hold it vertically. *C,* Grasp film and paper at lower center margin with left hand and, without bending or crimping, place it in exposure holder. *D,* Fold over top and side flaps of envelope. *E,* Fold end flap of envelope into place. *F,* Lower the holder cover and latch it. (Courtesy of Radiography Markets Division, Eastman Kodak Co.)

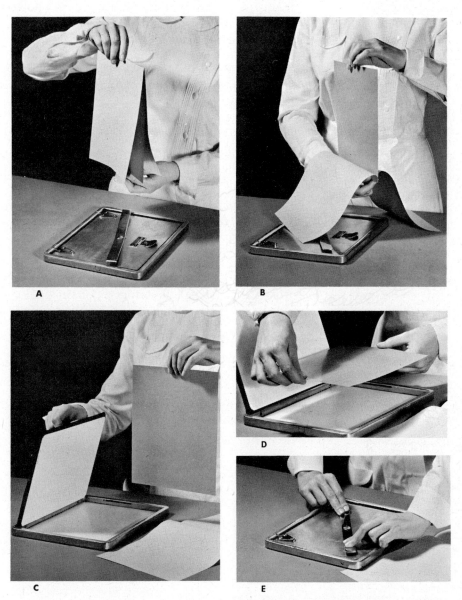

Figure 2-11 Loading cassette containing x-ray intensifying screens: *A,* Unlock cassette; remove film in its paper folder from box and hold it vertically with right hand. Separate film from paper with left hand and grasp lower edge of film between thumb and forefinger. *B,* With left hand still holding lower edge, turn film clockwise so paper falls away. *C,* Discard paper and raise cassette lid with right hand. *D,* Grasp film at center of lower edge with right hand, and, without bending it, lay it flat in cassette. *E,* Close cassette lid and lock it by spring lever. (Courtesy of Radiography Markets Division, Eastman Kodak Co.)

together at one end, with a metal clamp at the other end to lock the sides together when the holder is loaded and closed. One side has a lead backing to help absorb exit radiation; therefore the opposite side is placed nearest to the x-ray tube. Loading and unloading must be done in the dark room (Fig. 2–10). A "nonscreen" film, so called because it its more sensitive to x-rays than to fluorescent light, is used. The individual protective paper covering is left in place since it will not interfere with the exposure and since it provides extra protection against light exposure.

A cassette is a rigid framed film holder usually made of metal. The back side of the cassette is hinged for loading and is locked by metal clamps. The front side is the one placed towards the x-ray tube. Both sides have a built-in "intensifying screen" made of cardboard or a thin plastic sheet that is specially treated to give off a visible fluorescence of blue-green light when activated by x-rays. A screen film, sensitive to the fluorescent light as well as to the x-rays, is manufactured specifically for use with intensifying screens. This combination of fluorescent light and x-rays acting on the film shortens the exposure time and increases the image clarity. The film is loaded in the cassette in the dark room (Fig. 2–11). Although the paper covering is left in place when film holders are used, when a cassette is to be employed the cover must be removed (Fig. 2–12). Otherwise the covering will block the fluorescent effect just described.

When using either a film holder or cassette, small lead letters, "R" or "L" are necessary to indicate whether the film was held on the patient's right or left side. Because lead does not permit the passage of x-rays, the R and L will appear as white letters on the developed film. The letters are placed in one of the corners on the tube side of the holder or cassette and are held in place with tape.

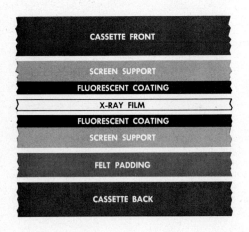

Figure 2–12 Diagram showing cross section of components of a loaded cassette. In use all elements should be in uniform contact. (Courtesy of Radiography Markets Division, Eastman Kodak Co.)

THE DARK ROOM

It is here that the films are processed—that is, developed, fixed, and washed. Because the films are sensitive to light, all light except that emitted from the safe light must be totally absent from the room, thus the term "dark room."

The processing tank is divided into three separate compartments. One is for the developer, one for the wash bath, and one for the fixer (Fig. 2–13). The wash bath is usually in the middle and is the largest of the three. It should have an overflow pipe so that fresh water can continually run into the tank during processing. A thermometer is placed in the wash bath, and the temperature of all three tanks is regulated by adjusting the flow of hot and cold water into the bath. Although the developing solution is usually on the left and the fixing solution on the right, this may not always be the arrangement. The important thing to know is which compartment has which solution.

Directions for preparing the developer and fixer can be found in the manufacturer's instructions on the packaged containers. The frequency with which you change solutions varies with the number of films being developed daily. A noticeable change in the quality of the radiograph (that is, if the image is becoming too faint after normal processing time) would seem to indicate that a change of solutions is necessary.

The time-temperature method of development is the procedure followed in most dental offices. This means that once the temperature of the solutions is established a specified length of time is needed for the films to be developed and fixed. Every attempt should be made to

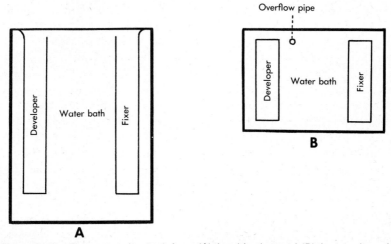

Figure 2–13   The processing tank from (A) the side view and (B) the top view, showing the developing and fixing compartments immersed in the water bath.

process films at the optimal temperature suggested by the manufacturer. Variations from the suggested temperature will necessitate changes in the developing and fixing times. If the solutions are warmer than optimum, the time is decreased; if they are cooler than optimum, the time is increased. However, the temperature should never exceed 85°, as the emulsion layer of the film will become very soft and difficult to handle.

Processing Procedure

The exposed film carries with it a latent image of the structures roentgenographed. Exposure of the film to x-rays or light causes a chemical change in the emulsion, and these changes will become evident when the film is immersed in the developing solution. In the developer those crystals of silver halide which have been exposed have the bromide portion of the crystal removed, leaving only metallic silver in the emulsion. This metallic silver is black in color and gives the developed film its black or gray areas. The gray tones are evident in areas where the crystals are incompletely or partially exposed. Here not all the silver halide has been reduced to metallic silver during development. If there are areas of the film that receive no radiation at all the silver bromide crystals remain unchanged during development. These areas appear white or clear on the completely processed film (Fig. 2–14).

When viewing an exposed film of the oral tissues it is readily seen that the dense tissues, such as the enamel of the teeth, bone, and metallic restorations, are the white areas. These lighter structures are called "radiopaque" because they are of a density capable of absorbing most x-rays and do not permit them to reach the film. This is in contrast to the darkest areas of the film. Here the x-rays penetrate the tissues with little or no resistance, and the silver bromide is completely changed to black metallic silver during development. These dark areas are known as "radiolucent" structures. Of course there is every gradation from white to black in these films, all dependent upon the degree of exposure of the film to the x-rays.

The number of x-rays used to expose the film determines the overall darkness of the processed radiograph. This degree of blackness is referred to as the density of the radiograph. Density is revealed when the film is held up to a light. An overexposed film will appear to be too dark (high density), whereas the underexposed film, which lacks density, will appear too light.

Image contrast, on the other hand, is the difference in densities of adjacent shadows recorded on the film. The greater the difference in densities between two adjacent structures, the greater or higher the

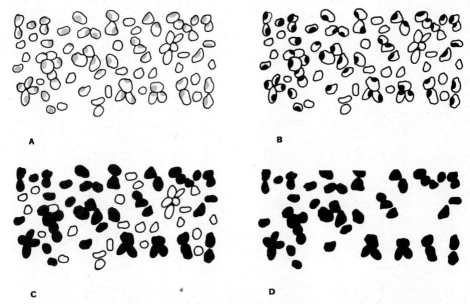

Figure 2–14 Diagrams of processing action in x-ray film emulsion. *A,* Schematic distribution of silver halide grains. The gray areas indicate latent image produced by exposure. *B,* Partial development begins to produce metallic silver (black) in exposed grains. *C,* Development completed. *D,* Unexposed silver grains have been removed by fixing. (Courtesy of Radiography Markets Division, Eastman Kodak Co.)

image contrast. "Short scale" contrast means that there is a predominance of black and white images with very few shades of gray intermixed. "Long scale" contrast will reveal different shades of gray with very few black or white shadows. Contrast is basically a function of the KVP. The lower the KVP, the greater the image contrast. Neither "long" nor "short" scale contrast is superior. It is a matter of the dentist's preference. However, most dentists feel that "short scale" contrast is better for diagnosing interproximal caries.

Before processing, all films must be identified in some manner to avoid confusing them with films of other patients. One method is to place the film packets in an envelope marked with the patient's name as soon as they are exposed. In the dark room make a notation on the envelope of the number of the film rack on which the films have been placed. Upon completion of the drying time the developed films are put back into the envelope until they are mounted.

When you are ready to process the films be certain that all lights except the safe light are turned off. Extraoral films are removed from the film holder or cassette and placed on large film racks. If you have film packets they must be stripped of their outer protective wrapping. Remove the films from the packets, holding the edges of the film rather than the flat surfaces, and place them on a film rack (Fig. 2–15).

The films are then put into the developing solution which contains

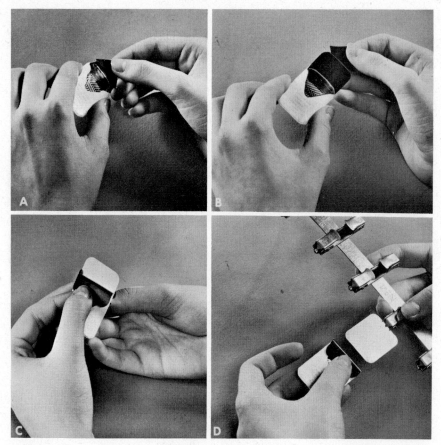

Figure 2–15 Preparation of intraoral film for processing: *A,* Pull up and out on the black tab to tear open the top of the packet. *B,* Pull on the black tab until about half of the black paper is out of the packet. *C,* Hold the black paper away from the film. *D,* Clip film on hanger, one film to a clip. (Courtesy of Radiography Markets Division, Eastman Kodak Co.)

either elon or hydroquinone as the developing agent. This solution also contains (1) sodium sulfite, which prevents the developer solution from oxidizing in the presence of air, (2) sodium carbonate, which activates the developing agents and maintains the alkalinity of the developer, and (3) potassium bromide, which inhibits the developer from acting on the unexposed silver salts. At this time the silver halide crystals which have been exposed have the halide portion of the crystal removed, leaving only the black metallic silver in the emulsion. However, if the film is left in the developing solution beyond the specified length of time, even those crystals which received no activation from x-radiation will lose the bromide portion. This will give the film an overall appearance of being too dark.

After the film has been in the developer for the correct length of time, it is thoroughly rinsed in the wash bath by several rapid immersions of the film rack. As much of the developer as possible should be removed from the film while it is in the wash bath. This will delay contamination of the fixing solution by the developer.

Now place the film in the fixing solution which contains either sodium or ammonia thiosulfate. This chemical dissolves and removes the underdeveloped silver halide from the film emulsion which clears the film so that the black or darker images become more perceptible. Other chemicals in the fixing solution are (1) sodium sulphite, which acts as a preservative preventing a breakdown of the chemicals, (2) acetic acid, which helps the other fixing agents to function properly (the acid also neutralizes the alkaline developer that may cling to the emulsion), and (3) potassium alum, which hardens the emulsion making it durable for handling of film. Before being placed in the fixing solution, the film still contained unchanged (unexposed) silver halide crystals. These unaltered crystals are removed by the fixing solution, thus completing the developing process. If a film is removed from the fixer prematurely you will see black and yellowish-brown areas which contain the unexposed silver bromide crystals. The "clearing time" is the length of time necessary to completely remove these crystals, leaving a clear area on the film. A film should always be left in the fixer for twice the length of time needed for clearing. The additional time is necessary to allow hardening of the emulsion, thus permitting you to carefully handle the film without damaging it. The usual length of time in the fixing solution is 10 minutes.

After removal from the fixer, the film is again placed in the wash bath to remove all the agents used to process the film. The final wash time usually takes 20 to 30 minutes when there is constant flow of fresh water into the bath. A longer period of washing time will be needed if the water is not circulating.

After the wash bath the films are hung up to dry or are placed in a dryer. When completely dry they are ready for mounting.

A recent advancement in film processing is the automatic film processor. There are several different brands on the market, all of which function basically on the same principle. Once the film is stripped of its protective wrapping it is inserted in a slot, picked up by revolving rollers, and carried through the respective tanks (developer, fixer, and so on). In a matter of 2 to 6 minutes the film is emitted from the drying chamber ready for mounting. In another type of processor the films are stationary in the unit and the respective solutions are dispensed separately by timing devices.

An option with most units is the daylight loader, a protective cloth with elastic cuffs that lets you strip the film and place it in the processor without being in a darkroom. This easily adapts to chairside processing if this is preferred.

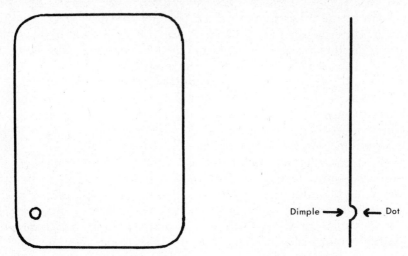

Dimple →　← Dot

Figure 2-16 Front and side views of film.

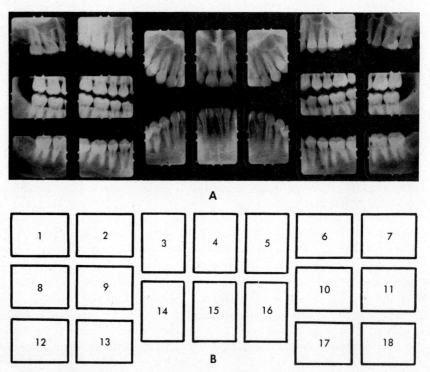

Figure 2-17 *A* and *B*, A full series of mounted x-rays. Films 1 through 7 are of the maxillary arch: (1) third molar region, (2) bicuspid-molar region, (3) cuspid region, (4) central-lateral incisor region, (5) cuspid region, (6) bicuspid-molar region, (7) third molar region. Films 8 through 11 are bite-wing exposures. Films 12 through 18 are of the mandibular arch: (12) third molar region, (13) bicuspid-molar region, (14) cuspid region, (15) central-lateral incisor region, (16) cuspid region, (17) bicuspid-molar region, (18) third molar region.

If there is a disadvantage to using these units it would be that the radiograph might be slightly fogged because of the special high-speed chemicals used and the higher temperatures of the solutions needed to speed up the processing time. This fogging, if present, is usually not that objectionable when weighed against the advantages.

Film Mounting

The types of mounts and mounting procedures used are a matter of the dentist's preference. There is a mark on the film which is called the "dimple" or the "dot," depending upon which side of the film you are viewing (Fig. 2–16). If the films are mounted so that they coincide with the teeth as you look at the patient's teeth, the dot side of the film should face you as you view the mounted x-rays. The alternate method would be viewing the films from the lingual side of the teeth; in this case the dimple side of the film would be facing you (Fig. 2–17).

REMINDERS

1. Maintain firm pressure on activating button until exposure time is complete.
2. The plain white surface of the film always faces the x-ray tube when placing intraoral or extraoral films.
3. For films that are to be placed in a permanent record, do not "short cut" the processing steps. The exposed film must be developed, fixed, and washed exactly as directed.
4. When stripping the film make sure your fingers are dry. Avoid finger-printing the emulsion.

3

ANATOMICAL LANDMARKS

God gives every bird its food, but He does
not throw it into the nest.

J. G. Holland

Anatomical landmarks are those normal structures and areas which appear in a routine series of radiographs. However, these structures will not appear with the same clarity for all patients. In one case a certain landmark may be outstanding, whereas in another it may be barely discernible, if at all.

Some structures are always visible in dental radiographs, regardless of the specific area exposed. Except, of course, in the endentulous patient, the teeth themselves are one such structure (Fig. 3–1). As viewed on a radiograph a normal tooth has an outer, whiter layer surrounding the crown of the tooth. This is the enamel covering of the crown (1),*and it is the most dense tissue in the human body. Just underneath the enamel is the dentin (2). This middle layer of the tooth extends from the crown into the root. Dentin is not as hard or dense as enamel, although it is still radiopaque. The root of the tooth is covered by a very thin layer of cementum, less dense than dentin, and therefore usually not discernible. The innermost portion is the pulp canal, which contains nerves and blood vessels (3). It is radiolucent and appears dark in a radiograph because it is composed of soft tissue through which x-rays readily penetrate to the film. The canal extends from the crown of the tooth through the root to the root apex.

The supporting structures of the teeth are also evident on all radiographs. The maxilla in the upper arch and the mandible in the lower arch are the bones which support the teeth. They are made up of two types of bone. The cortical bone, known as the lamina dura (4), appears white or radiopaque because of its dense structure. This is the bone

---

*Parenthesized numbers in this chapter refer to labeled parts of the illustration under discussion.

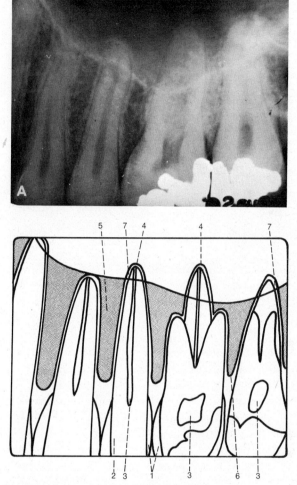

Figure 3–1 *A,* Radiograph of the maxillary posterior teeth showing common structures seen in other periapical radiographs. *B,* Diagrammatic sketch of the radiograph used to point out the different structures. (1) Enamel, (2) dentin, (3) pulp canal (nerves and blood vessels), (4) lamina dura, (5) cancellous bone, (6) alveolar crest, (7) periodontal membrane space.

that immediately surrounds and supports the teeth. The remaining bone is much less dense in its composition, having marrow spaces within its structural make-up. This is cancellous bone (5). It has a spongy or cancellous consistency and appears less radiopaque than the cortical bone. The alveolar bone of the maxilla or mandible is that part of the bone from which the teeth erupt and by which they are maintained in position. It is made up of both cortical and cancellous bone. The edge of this bone is referred to as the alveolar crest (6). Between the root of the tooth and the lamina dura is a fine radiolucent line which is the ligamentous attachment of the tooth to the bone. This is

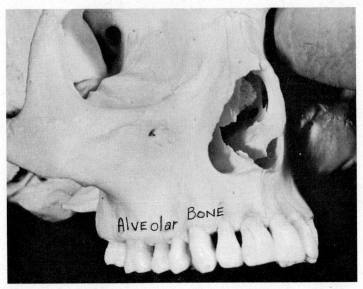

Figure 3-2 The alveolar bone from which the teeth erupt and by which they are maintained in position.

called the periodontal membrane space (7). Figure 3–2 is a photograph of a skull showing the area of bone on the maxilla that is termed alveolar bone.

The series of radiographs used in the discussion that follows are periapical films; that is, they show the entire length of the tooth with emphasis on the root apex and supporting structures. In both the maxillary and mandibular arches the series begin with the anterior teeth, then proceed back to the cuspid region, the bicuspid region, and finally the molar region. To thoroughly acquaint you with the landmarks there is a description of each, a photograph of each, a radiograph of the area which demonstrates the respective landmarks, and a labeled diagrammatic explanation of each radiograph.

LANDMARKS OF THE MAXILLARY ARCH

Central-Lateral Incisor Region (Fig. 3–3). The oval or pear-shaped radiolucent area located between the apices of the central incisors is the anterior palatine or incisive canal foramen (opening) (1). The canal is composed of several smaller canals, and in some cases the openings of these smaller canals can be observed. Blood vessels and nerves occupy these canals. This landmark is not always prominent, the degree of clarity depending somewhat upon the thickness and density of the overlying bone. From the crest of the alveolar ridge between the cen-

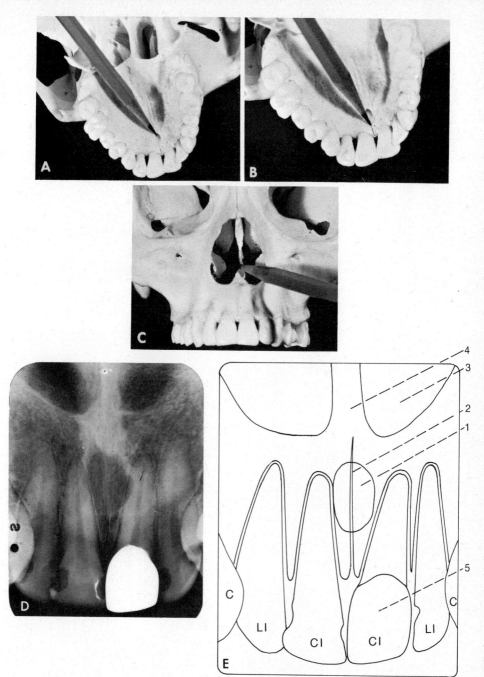

Figure 3-3 *A,* The tip of the pointer is on the anterior palatine canal foramen. The foramen is located on the palate just behind the central incisors and is the common orifice for other, smaller canals carrying blood vessels to the nose and mouth. Owing to the angle of the tube head when exposing the radiograph of this area, the foramen almost always appears slightly above or between the apices of the maxillary central incisors. *B,* The tip of the pointer is on the midpalatine suture. *C,* The pointer is placed within the nasal fossa. The nasal septum can also be seen as a partition within the fossa. *D* and *E,* Maxillary central-lateral incisor region showing (1) incisive canal foramen, (2) median palatine suture superimposed over the incisive canal foramen, (3) nasal fossa, (4) nasal septum, and (5) gold crown on the central incisor. Cl = central incisor; Ll = lateral incisor; C = cuspid.

tral incisors is a radiolucent line which extends posteriorly through the midline of the palate. This is the median palatine suture that marks the junction of the right and left palatine bones (2). Toward the upper portion of the radiograph are two radiolucent areas divided by a radiopaque band. These are the nasal fossae (3), which are air spaces,

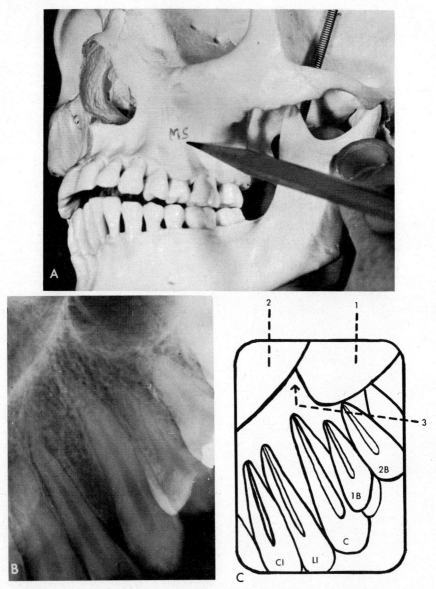

Figure 3–4 *A,* Maxillary sinus. The area marked MS is that portion of bone overlying the maxillary sinus. (Note: In some of the photographs of the skull in this and succeeding chapters you will see a screw and a spring. They are used to attach the mandible to the skull.) *B* and *C,* Maxillary cuspid region showing (1) maxillary sinus, (2) nasal fossa, and (3) "typical Y" formation of the maxillary sinus. 1B = first bicuspid; 2B = second bicuspid.

one on each side of the midline of the face, divided by the bony nasal septum (4).

Cuspid Region (Fig. 3–4).   With this exposure an important structure, the maxillary sinus (1), makes its appearance. Like the nasal fossae (2) it is an air space and appears as a radiolucent area. Where the anterosuperior (upper front) wall of the maxillary sinus joins with the floor of the nasal fossa there is formed what is known as the inverted "typical Y" of the maxillary sinus (3).

Bicuspid Region (Fig. 3–5).   This exposure shows the main por-

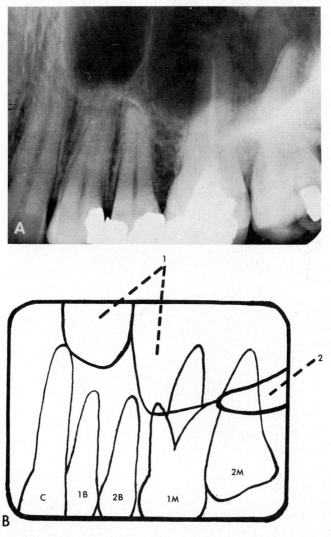

Figure 3–5   *A* and *B*, Maxillary bicuspid region showing (1) maxillary sinus divided by septum and (2) anterior portion of the zygomatic or malar bone. 1M = first molar; 2M = second molar.

tion of the maxillary sinus (1). Many radiographs will show the maxillary sinus extending into the alveolar ridge between the roots of the teeth. In areas where teeth are missing it may extend to the alveolar crest. The floor of the nasal cavity may also be visible above the supe-

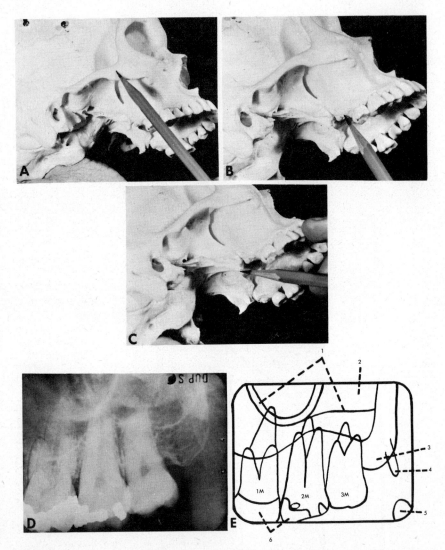

Figure 3–6 *A,* Zygomatic arch. This portion of the zygomatic arch forms the prominence of the cheek. *B,* The pointer is locating the maxillary tuberosity. It marks the posterior limit of the maxillary arch. *C,* The pointer is touching the hamular process, which is a hook- or pronglike bony structure located just posterior to the maxillary tuberosity. *D* and *E,* Maxillary molar region showing (1) zygomatic or malar bone, (2) zygomatic arch superimposed over maxillary sinus, (3) maxillary tuberosity, (4) hamular process, (5) coronoid process of the mandible, and (6) metallic restorations. 3M = third molar.

rior border of the sinus. The anterior portion of the zygomatic or malar bone usually appears in this exposure (2).

Molar Region (Fig. 3–6). The posterior border of the maxillary sinus is now present. A prominent landmark is the zygomatic or malar bone which forms the prominence of the cheek (1). Radiographically speaking, the zygomatic bone appears as a U-shaped radiopacity usually found in the apical region of the first and second molar and usually superimposed over the molar root tips. When prominent, the zygomatic arch appears as a radiopaque band extending posteriorly from the zygomatic bone (2). Other radiopaque structures seen in this exposure are the maxillary tuberosity (3) and the hamular process

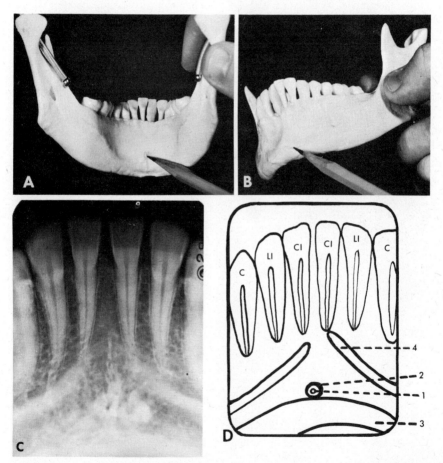

Figure 3–7   *A,* The pointer is touching the genial tubercles. Two of each are located on either side of the midline. *B,* The pointer is touching the mental process, a thickening of bone on the anterior labial surface of the mandible. *C* and *D,* Mandibular central-lateral incisor region showing (1) lingual foramen, (2) genial tubercles, (3) inferior border of the mandible, and (4) mental process or ridge.

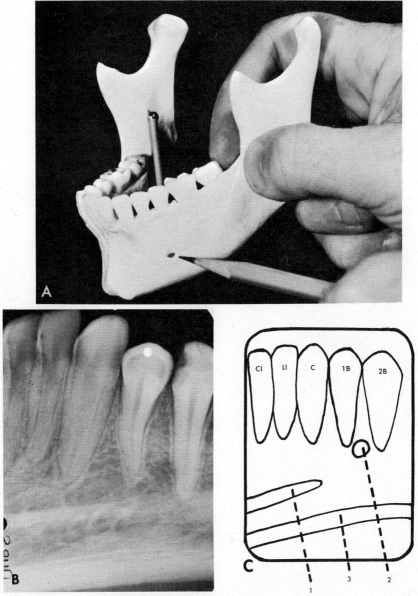

Figure 3–8 *A,* The pointer is locating the mental foramen on the outer surface of the mandible. *B* and *C,* Mandibular cuspid region showing (1) mental process, (2) mental foramen, and (3) inferior border of the mandible.

which serves as a tendinous attachment for muscle fibers (4), both of which are composed mostly of cancellous bone. The coronoid process of the mandible (5), serving as a point of muscle attachment, is usually visible also.

LANDMARKS OF THE MANDIBULAR ARCH

Central-Lateral Incisor Region (Fig. 3–7).   Just beneath the apices of the central incisors is a small radiolucent circular area, the lingual foramen (1). The foramen is surrounded by four bony spines for muscle

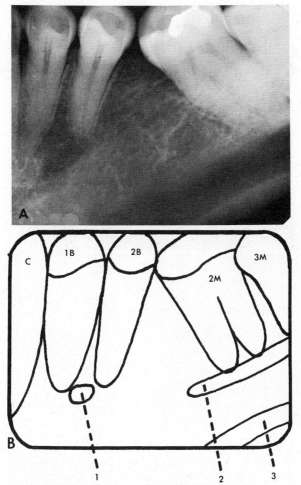

Figure 3–9 *A* and *B,* Mandibular bicuspid region showing (1) mental foramen, (2) mylohyoid line or ridge, and (3) inferior border of the mandible.

attachment, the genial tubercles (2). These tubercles are in such close apposition to each other that when viewed in a radiograph of this area they have the appearance of a radiopaque circle. These two structures are located on the lingual side and near the inferior border of the mandible (3). The ridge or thickening of bone located below the apices of

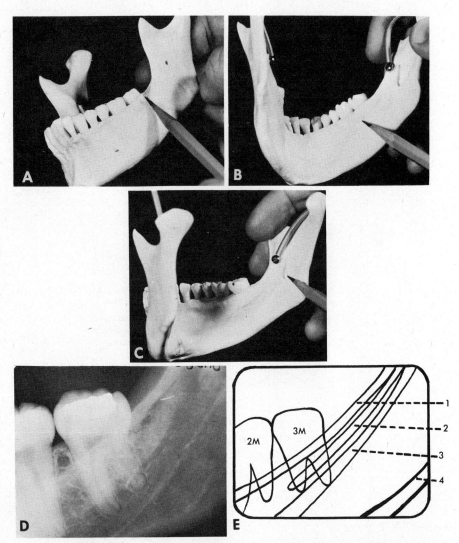

Figure 3–10 *A,* The pointer is placed on the external oblique line, which is the continuation of the anterior border on the outer surface of the mandible. This area of bone is usually very dense. *B,* The pointer is touching the internal oblique line, which is a ridge of condensed bone on the inner surface of the mandible. *C,* Mandibular canal. The pointer is locating the mandibular foramen on the inner surface of the mandible. From this point the canal travels anteriorly within the mandible to the mental foramen. *D* and *E,* Mandibular molar region showing (1) external oblique line or ridge, (2) internal oblique line or ridge, (3) mandibular canal, and (4) inferior border of the mandible.

the anterior teeth is the mental process or ridge (4). It is located on the labial side of the mandible. Being condensed bone, it appears as a radiopaque band extending from the midline of the mandible posteriorly to the bicuspid region.

Cuspid Region (Fig. 3–8).   No new landmark of any significance is present in this region. The posterior extension of the mental process (1), if prominent, will be seen. The mental foramen (2), which is the anterior orifice of the mandibular canal, normally lies just inferior to the apices of the bicuspids and may be seen, depending upon placement of the film for this exposure.

Bicuspid Region (Fig. 3–9).   The structure of importance in this region is the mental foramen (1). As viewed on the radiograph it appears as a small radiolucent area usually between and just inferior to the root apices of the bicuspids. At times it may be superimposed over the root apex of either bicuspid. In some radiographs you may be able

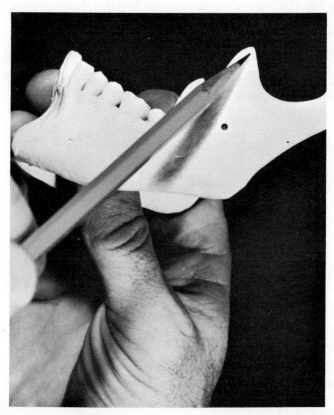

Figure 3–11 The pointer is locating the coronoid process of the mandible. When the patient opens his mouth, the coronoid process moves down to a point on or near the maxillary tuberosity. For this reason a portion of this structure is usually seen in a periapical radiograph of the maxillary third molar region.

to follow the mandibular canal with its blood vessels and nerves as it leads into the mental foramen. The mylohyoid line or ridge (2) may appear in this exposure. The inferior border of the mandible (3) is also visible.

Molar Region (Fig. 3–10). In this region there are two radiopaque lines. The upper line is a continuation of the ascending border of the mandible and usually terminates in the region of the first molar. This is the external oblique line or ridge which serves as an area for muscle attachment (1). Just inferior to this line is the radiopaque mylohyoid line or ridge (or the internal oblique line) (2), which is a thickening of the

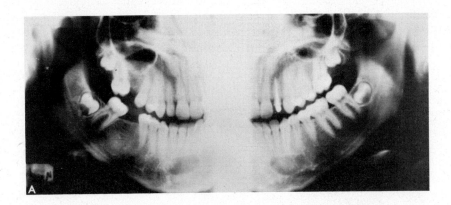

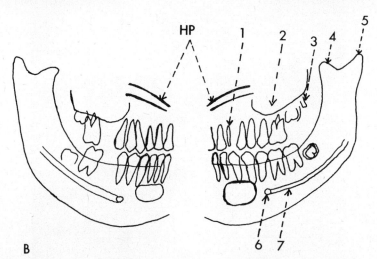

Figure 3–12 *A,* Panoramic radiograph of maxillary and mandibular arches. *B,* Schematic drawing of the above panoramic radiograph illustrating the respective anatomic landmarks: (1) endodontically treated tooth, (2) maxillary sinus, (3) hamulus, (4) coronoid process, (5) head of condyle, (6) mental foramen, (7) mandibular canal. Notice that all central and lateral incisors are seen on both sides of the midline of the film. A cyst is in evidence below the mandibular anterior teeth. HP = hard palate.

mandible for the attachment of the mylohyoid muscle. The mylohyoid line is usually visible for a greater distance anteriorly than the external oblique line. Also in this region is the mandibular canal (3), which usually appears outlined by a thin layer of cortical bone. This structure is a nutrient canal carrying nerves and blood vessels; hence it appears as a radiolucent canal in the region of the root apices of the molars. The orifice of the canal is the mandibular foramen. Although the coronoid process is part of the mandible it is not seen in periapical radiographs of the mandible. Because of its position it is seen in periapical radiographs of the maxillary third molar region (Figs. 3–11 and 3–12).

REMINDERS

1. The three radiolucent structures usually seen in the maxillary central incisor exposure that are not associated with the teeth are the incisive canal foramen, nasal fossae, and the midpalatine suture.
2. In the maxillary cuspid exposure you will usually see two large radiolucent landmarks, the nasal fossa, and the maxillary sinus.
3. The radiopaque structure often superimposed over the root tips of the maxillary first and second molars is the malar bone.
4. The coronoid process is seen only in the maxillary third molar periapical exposure.
5. An important radiolucent landmark usually located at or between the apices of the mandibular bicuspid teeth is the mental foramen. It may be superimposed over the apex of either one of the bicuspids and can be mistaken for an abscess.
6. When the external and internal oblique lines are seen together on the same radiograph, the external oblique line occupies the superior position.

4

THE BISECTION OF THE ANGLE TECHNIQUE

Do a little more each day than you think you possibly can.

Lowell Thomas

THE CASE OF THE EQUILATERAL TRIANGLE

Because of irregularities in the make-up of the oral tissues, the film cannot always be placed parallel to the teeth being radiographed. When the teeth and the film are not parallel with one another, the x-ray may produce a shadow on the film that is either shorter or longer than the teeth themselves. To obtain a shadow equal in length to the teeth, the bisection of the angle technique is used.

The success of this technique is based on the theory that if two triangles have a common side and two equal angles they are equal triangles. In Figure 4–1 the triangle ABC is divided into two triangles by the common side XY. The line XY bisects the angle at B, forming two triangles, ABD and BCD. The angles at B are made equal by the bisecting line XY. The bisecting line also forms two 90-degree angles where it joins side AC. From this we see that the two triangles thus formed each have two equal angles and a common side; therefore they are equal.

We can apply this principle to shadow casting. When you take an x-ray of a tooth you are casting a shadow of that tooth onto the film. In Figure 4–2 the light source comes from point L in the arc MN. The light is directed toward the object, casting a shadow of that object onto the film. When the light comes from point L, the shadow caused by the object is of the same length as the object. If the light source is lowered to point P in the arc, the shadow will be much longer than the actual length of the object. When the light source is positioned at point Q in the arc the length of the shadow is less than the length of the object.

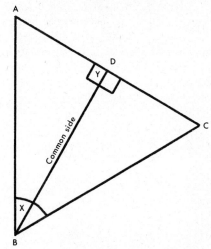

Figure 4-1

Let us now draw a line XY that bisects the angle formed by the object and the film. Notice that when the light crosses XY, it forms an angle of 90 degrees. *This last sentence is the key to the bisection of the angle technique.* In this diagram you can see that two equal triangles have been formed by the bisecting line XY, with side AB being equal to side A'B'.

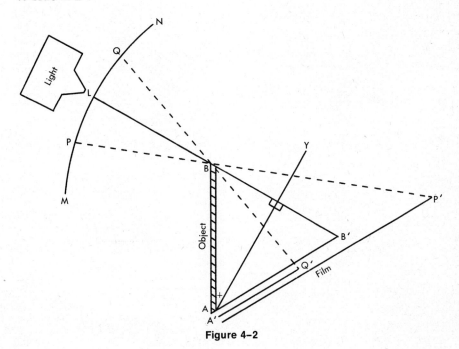

Figure 4-2

In the patient's mouth the tooth (or teeth) becomes the object (Fig. 4–3A). Erect an imaginary line that bisects the angle formed by the tooth and the film, directing the central ray to the center of the film and perpendicular (at a 90-degree angle) to the imaginary line. If this is

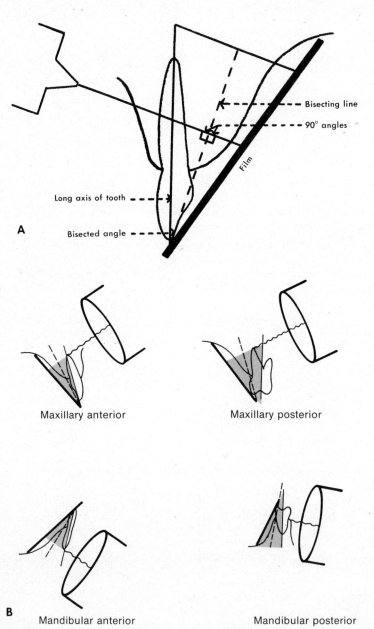

Bisecting line

90° angles

Film

Long axis of tooth

A   Bisected angle

Maxillary anterior   Maxillary posterior

B   Mandibular anterior   Mandibular posterior

Figure 4–3 *A*, Triangle superimposed over tooth and oral tissues. *B*, Shaded areas represent the angle formed by the teeth and film that is bisected to form two equilateral triangles.

done correctly you will have created two equal triangles in the patient's mouth, the length of the shadow of the tooth recorded on the film being equal to the actual length of the tooth (or teeth) being radiographed. Figure 4–3*B* demonstrates the bisection of the angle principle in the four segments of the arches.

PLACEMENT OF FILM AND TUBE HEAD

The placement of the film so that it is centered over the area of interest is of prime importance when using this technique. As an aid to correct film placement, a guide line lightly drawn on the film packet has proved to be an invaluable aid.

All periapical films to be used in exposing the anterior regions (incisors and cuspids) of both arches have a line drawn vertically through the long axis of each film dividing it into right and left halves (Fig. 4–4*A*). For films used to expose the posterior teeth, in which the film is placed horizontally in the mouth, the line is drawn through the center of the film perpendicular to its long axis (Fig. 4–4*B*).

To place the film correctly it must be centered over a specific tooth or area. Since the guide line marks the center of the film, by placing the film so that the guide line falls on the specific tooth or area required for that particular exposure, you know you have centered the film correctly. The guide line aids mainly in centering the film anteroposteriorly (horizontally). Vertical placement of the film is ⅛ to ¼ inch above or below the occlusal line, depending upon the arch being examined. The exact film placement and the teeth or areas over which the guide line should fall are noted in the following chapters under the descriptions of the various techniques. It should be noted that with some patients film placement as directed cannot be performed correctly

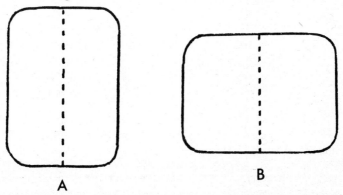

Figure 4–4 Guide lines for anteroposterior film placement for *(A)* anterior region and *(B)* posterior region.

owing to anatomical restrictions. When this condition arises, use your own judgment in placing the film as nearly correctly as possible.

In addition to film placement you must also become familiar with the different angulations of the tube head. The vertical angulations, that is the up and down angulation of the cone tip, will be deviations from a line parallel with the floor (Fig. 4–5). All angulations above this parallel line are called plus vertical angulations; all angulations below this line are minus vertical angulations. The maxillary arch is exposed to x-ray with the cone tip above the occlusal line (0 degrees horizontally); therefore plus (+) vertical angulations are used. The radiograph of the mandibular arch is taken from below this line so that minus (−) vertical angulations are used.

The horizontal angulation is the second phase in adjusting the tube head. It refers to the sideways placement of the cone tip. The horizontal placement is not governed by definite numbered angulations, owing to the great variance in arch forms and position of the teeth. The one rule to follow is to make sure that the central rays pass through the teeth parallel to the proximal surfaces (the surfaces of a tooth which come in contact with adjacent teeth of the same arch) (Fig. 4–6). If the

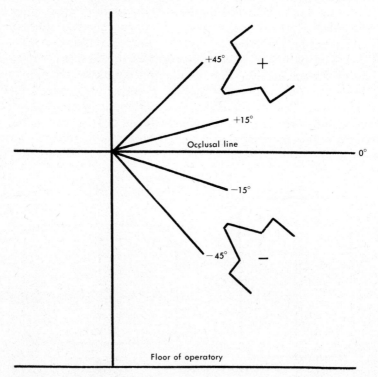

Figure 4–5 Side view showing vertical angulations with occlusal line parallel to the floor.

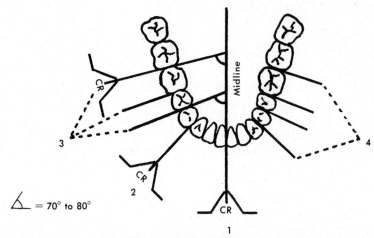

Figure 4–6 Occlusal view of the teeth showing horizontal angulations for (1) incisor exposure, (2) cuspid exposure, and (3) posterior exposures, and showing (4) the proximal surfaces.

central rays are not parallel, the resultant image will show overlapping of the proximal surfaces. Although there are no specific angulations for posterior exposures, in the majority of patients you will find that the central rays pass parallel to the proximal surfaces at an angle of 70 to 80 degrees from the midline (Fig. 4–6).

In the next two chapters you will note that a vertical angulation is given for each periapical exposure. It is most important that you understand that these angulations will prove correct for the average patient only. The correct way to use the bisection of the angle technique is to do just that—bisect the angle formed by the tooth and film as previously explained. It will be to your advantage to free yourself as quickly as possible from these preset vertical angulations. No two patients have exactly the same oral anatomy. In a patient with a high palatal vault, the angle formed by the film and tooth would be much less than that in an average patient. Obviously, the vertical angulations required for the same exposure would differ.

TAKING THE RADIOGRAPH

When using the bisection of the angle technique there are certain steps or rules that should be studied and committed to memory. A thorough knowledge of the principles involved and the rules to follow will give you the confidence and know-how to obtain highly accurate radiographs of your patients. The rules are listed in order of their application to the patient. As you study them, form a mental image of yourself going through the procedure.

As you seat the patient, ask him to remove any partial or complete dentures, removable bridges, eyeglasses, and so on, as these may be superimposed over the area of interest when viewing the resultant radiograph.

Adjust the headrest of the dental chair so that the arch to be exposed to the x-ray beam is parallel to the floor when the mouth is open.

Many patients find it awkward and uncomfortable to have a film packet placed in their mouths. To alleviate some of the discomfort and to make the film more adaptable to the patient's oral tissues, soften the film packet by lightly bending the corners between your thumb and index finger. Be careful not to crease the film.

Place the film in the patient's mouth, centering it gently over the area of interest (teeth, ridge) so as not to irritate the sensitive oral tissues. Do not slide it into position.

Instruct the patient to hold the film in this precise position, using his thumb for all maxillary exposures and his index finger for all mandibular exposures. To prevent excess bending of the film at the root apex have the patient apply finger pressure at the junction of the tooth crown and gum line (Fig. 4–7). If for some reason the patient is unable to do this, the use of one of the many types of film holders is necessary. When a film holder is used, the angle of the film is almost always changed from the angle it assumes under finger pressure and the film

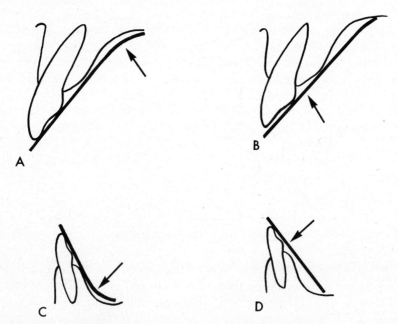

Figure 4–7 Arrows indicate finger pressure holding film in place. For maxillary arch: *A,* Incorrect—finger pressure too high. *B,* Correct—finger pressure at crown-gingival junction. For mandibular arch: *C,* Incorrect—finger pressure too low. *D,* Correct—finger pressure at crown-gingival junction.

becomes more parallel with the teeth. Therefore a reduction in the vertical angulation is required to compensate for this change. The horizontal angulation is not altered.

To reduce the tendency for patients to gag, the radiographic procedure should start with the upper central incisors. By starting here and working posteriorly toward the third molar area with each successive exposure, the patient's palate becomes conditioned to the film placement.

When the film is maintained in its correct position by the patient, you are free to adjust the tube head to the correct vertical and horizontal angulations. The cone tip should always lightly contact the patient's skin for each intraoral exposure. This assures you of proper density and contrast in the films when viewing a complete series.

Make sure that the central ray is directed toward the center of the film for each exposure.

Take your position behind a wall or protective shield, and press the activating button. Keep pressure on the button until the unit automatically shuts off.

CARE OF THE X-RAY UNIT

In order to keep the x-ray unit in good operating condition, these suggestions should be followed.

A. Do not force the unit arm to be overextended or to be pressed into an overly compact position.

B. When you are finished using the x-ray unit, do not leave the arm of the unit extended over the chair. The tube head is quite heavy and will exert undue stress on the unit arm. Over a period of time, this will result in drifting of the tube head after you have positioned it for an exposure. Place the unit arm compactly when not in use.

C. Do not allow the tube head to make contact with the wall or any other piece of equipment, as this will tend to loosen the seal, thereby allowing the oil or gas coolant surrounding the x-ray tube to leak out.

D. If you need to readjust the x-ray unit for different MA and KVP readings, you may have to press the activating button several times for trial adjustments before obtaining the desired readings. Always allow sufficient time between each reading to ensure adequate cooling of the tube (approximately 5 seconds). Rapid firing of the tube produces a tremendous heat build-up which may result in heat spots or pitting of the tube target.

E. When the x-ray unit will not be used for a length of time, such as an afternoon away from the office or overnight, turn off the electric current at the off-on switch, usually located on the cabinet of the unit.

REMINDERS

1. All periapical film placements for anterior teeth should be placed with the long axis of the film in a vertical position. For posterior teeth, the film is placed with the long axis in a horizontal position.
2. Adjust the vertical angulation to record accurate lengths of the teeth on the film image. Failure to do so will produce images of the teeth that are too long or too short.
3. Adjust the horizontal angulation to record open contacts between the teeth. Failure to do so will produce an image with one tooth superimposed or overlapped with an adjacent tooth.
4. If the film isn't placed correctly, do not expose it. A retake with its added patient exposure will be necessary to make the corrections.
5. Aim the central ray of the x-ray beam to the center of the film. This will ensure the complete overall exposure of the film.
6. You must always press the activating button firmly until the exposure time is completed.

5

EXPOSING PERIAPICAL FILMS OF THE MAXILLARY ARCH

Skill to do comes of doing.

Emerson

A full series of x-rays is made up of a number of films showing the teeth and the condition of their supporting structures. No definite number of periapical radiographs comprises the full series; but a minimum of 14 films is needed to adequately survey both arches. Bite-wing exposures should accompany these periapical films to make the radiographic examination complete. The seven films of the maxillary arch are the central and lateral incisor exposure, and both right and left exposures of the cuspid, bicuspid-molar, and third molar areas.

THE CENTRAL AND LATERAL INCISOR EXPOSURE (Fig. 5–1)

A. Make the maxillary arch parallel to the floor by adjusting the headrest.

B. Place the film vertically in the patient's mouth, centering it over the contact point between the two central incisors.

C. The lower edge of the film should be parallel to and extend 1/8 inch below the edges of the teeth.

D. Instruct the patient to hold the film in this exact position with either thumb, exerting light but firm pressure against the inside or tongue surface of the crowns. Check again to see that the maxillary arch is parallel with the floor.

E. Bisect the angle to establish the correct vertical angulation (approximately +40 degrees).

F. The horizontal angulation is established by directing the central rays through the midline of the patient's face.

G. Always point the central ray to the center of the film.

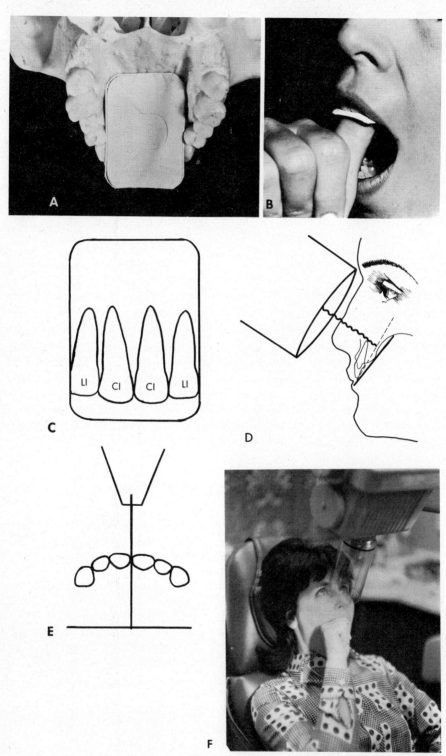

See legend on opposite page.

THE CUSPID EXPOSURE (Figs. 5–2 through 5–6)

A. Make the maxillary arch parallel to the floor.

B. Place the film vertically in the patient's mouth, centering it over the cuspid (Fig. 5–2A and B).

C. The lower edge of the film should be parallel to the occlusal line of the teeth and should extend 1/8 inch below the cusp tip of the cuspid (Fig. 5–2C).

D. Instruct the patient to hold the film in this exact position, with the thumb opposite the side on which the film is placed. Check again to see that the maxillary arch is parallel with the floor.

E. Bisect the angle to establish the correct vertical angulation (approximately +40 degrees). The vertical angulation of the cuspid exposure almost always approximates that used for the central and lateral incisor exposure (Fig. 5–2D).

F. The horizontal angulation for this exposure is one of the more difficult ones to learn. As seen in Figure 5–2E, the circled 1 represents the point where the edge of the cone touches the patient when exposing the central incisor. The circled 2 represents the point where the edge of the cone touches the patient for the cuspid exposure. For the best possible view of the cuspid, the central ray is directed through the contact point between the cuspid and the first bicuspid (Fig. 5–2F). If the cone is not swung around posteriorly to this position after taking the central and lateral exposure, there will be too much overlap between the cuspid and the first bicuspid (Fig. 5–3A and B). Therefore once you have exposed the central and lateral incisor exposure, get into the habit of swinging the tube head around to a point which closely approximates the horizontal angulation used for the bicuspid exposure (Fig. 5–3C and D). This may seem rather odd to you since the cuspid is considered an anterior tooth, but if you follow this "swing around" procedure you will be pleased with the results.

G. Always point the central ray to the center of the film.

Alternative Film Placement for Cuspid Exposure

Owing to the many variations in the shape of palates there may be difficulty in placing the film high enough and parallel with the occlusal

---

Figure 5–1 Central and lateral incisor exposure. *A*, Position of film over teeth on skull. *B*, Patient holding film in position. *C*, Diagram of teeth in relation to the film. *D*, Illustration of bisection of the angle principle. *E*, Horizontal angulation. *F*, Position of patient, film, and cone for exposure.

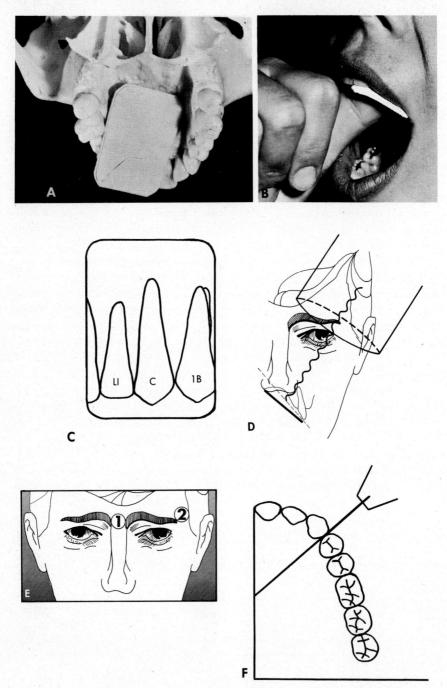

Figure 5–2 Cuspid exposure: *A*, Position of film over teeth on skull. *B*, Patient holding film in position. *C*, Diagram of teeth in relation to the film. *D*, Illustration of bisection of the angle principle. *E*, Points where cone touches patient. *F*, Horizontal angulation.

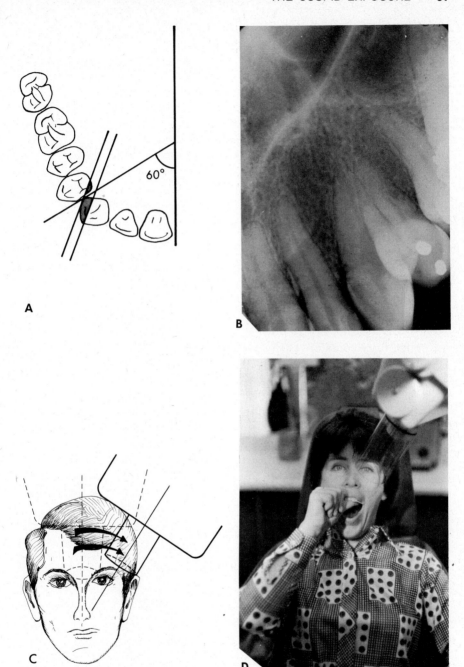

Figure 5–3 Cuspid exposure. *A* and *B,* Many problems can be eliminated when exposing the maxillary cuspid if you will place the tube head so that the horizontal angulation is moved to approximately 60 from the midline. By so doing you will produce a radiograph without overlap of adjacent teeth. If you direct the central rays into the labial surface of the cuspid (double lines in *A*), the resultant radiograph will have overlapped images of the distal of the cuspid with the first bicuspid (*B*). *C,* Swinging the tube head around for cuspid exposure. *D,* Position of patient, film, and cone for exposure.

line. This is especially true when the patient has a narrow palate. If you have tried to place the film in the standard position as described above and find that the upper anterior corner of the film impinges on the opposite side of the palate, DO NOT FORCE THE FILM TO BEND UP INTO THE PALATE when attempting to place it high enough.

When this problem arises the "oblique" film placement should be used. As the upper anterior corner of the film makes contact with the palate or teeth on the opposite side, slide that corner posteriorly (maintaining contact with the palate or teeth) and rotate the lower portion of the film anteriorly to a point where it contacts one or both incisal edges of the central incisors (Fig. 5–4A through G). It is important not to rotate the film beyond the oblique position, for this will cause it to become too horizontal, resulting in the apex of the cuspid root being projected off the edge of the film.

As complicated as this may seem, the oblique placement of the film is a simple movement. Just read the steps over and correlate each with the drawing until the procedure becomes familiar. The cuspid is the only tooth of major concern in this exposure, and the oblique film placement satisfactorily covers this tooth and its supporting structures. However, every attempt should be made first to place the film in a standard edge-to-edge manner (Fig. 5–5A and B).

Some dental arches are so narrow that they almost come to a point through the anterior region. Such arches are described as "V"-shaped. With this condition it is all but impossible to place the film accurately in either the standard or oblique position, so we use the cross-arch position. Place the film on top of the occlusal surfaces of the teeth in vertical alignment with the cuspid to be radiographed (Fig. 5–6). Position the tube head and the cone in the same manner as for the other two positions. The vertical angle will be higher than that routinely seen, owing to the increased angle between the long axis of the cuspid and the film.

BICUSPID-MOLAR EXPOSURE (Fig. 5–7)

A. Make the maxillary arch parallel to the floor.

B. Place the film horizontally in the patient's mouth, with the anterior edge of the film lying over the anterior half of the cuspid.

C. The lower edge of the film should be parallel to the occlusal line of the bicuspid and molar teeth, extending ¼ inch below that line.

D. Instruct the patient to hold the film in this exact position, with the thumb opposite the side on which the film is placed. Check again to see if the maxillary arch is parallel with the floor.

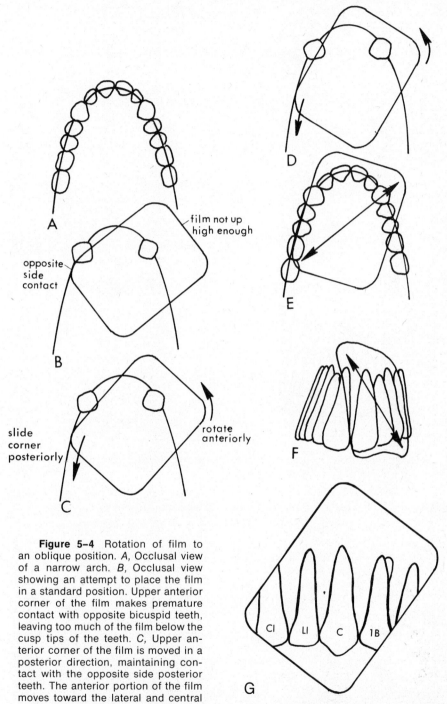

Figure 5–4 Rotation of film to an oblique position. *A*, Occlusal view of a narrow arch. *B*, Occlusal view showing an attempt to place the film in a standard position. Upper anterior corner of the film makes premature contact with opposite bicuspid teeth, leaving too much of the film below the cusp tips of the teeth. *C*, Upper anterior corner of the film is moved in a posterior direction, maintaining contact with the opposite side posterior teeth. The anterior portion of the film moves toward the lateral and central incisors. *D*, Continuing movement described in *C*. *E*, Film is now up high enough to record the cuspid in a corner-to-corner direction on the film. *F*, Front view of the oblique film position. *G*, Position of cuspid on the film.

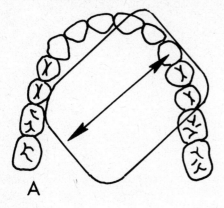

A

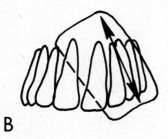

B

Figure 5–5 Standard edge-to-edge film position. *A*, Occlusal view. *B*, Front view.

E. Bisect the angle to establish the correct vertical angulation (approximately +30 to +35 degrees).

F. The horizontal angulation is established by directing the central rays parallel to the proximal surfaces of the bicuspid and molar teeth.

G. Always point the central rays to the center of the film.

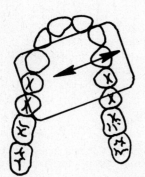

Figure 5–6 Cross-arch film position.

THE THIRD MOLAR EXPOSURE (Fig. 5–8)

A. Make the maxillary arch parallel to the floor.

B. Place the film horizontally in the patient's mouth, centering it over the third molar. (If the molar is impacted, center the film over the third molar region.)

C. The lower edge of the film should be parallel to and even with the cusp tips of the first and second molars. Because of the elevated position of the third molar (more elevated if the tooth is impacted), the film must assume a higher position on the palate so that an adequate exposure may be obtained.

D. Instruct the patient to hold the film in this exact position, with the thumb or index finger opposite the side on which the film is placed. When placing the film for this exposure, any tendency for the patient to gag may be alleviated by treating the palate with a topical anesthetic. Check to see that the maxillary arch is parallel to the floor.

E. Bisect the angle to establish the correct vertical angulation. Since the film lies in a more horizontal or flatter position in conforming to the posterior palatal region, the plus vertical angulation may be as high as +45 to +50 degrees after bisecting the angle.

F. The horizontal angulation is established by directing the central rays through the third molar region parallel to the proximal surfaces of the molar teeth.

G. Always point the central ray to the center of the film.

Note: There is a greater volume of bone in this region, tending to absorb more of the x-rays. To compensate for this, a slight increase in the time exposure may be necessary, according to the dentist's wishes.

Consult film manufacturer's instructions for dial settings and exposure time.

Film, patient, and cone tip positioning when using the pointed plastic cone for maxillary periapical exposures are shown in Figure 5–9.

THE BITE-BLOCK FILM HOLDER

When taking the radiographs described in this chapter, all films are held in position by having the patient use finger pressure against the back of the film. Digital retention of the film has always been used by most dentists and their staff simply because this is the way they were taught and it has proved to be practical and satisfactory.

An alternative method is the use of a bite-block film holder. There are many types of bite blocks on the market today, all of which have proved satisfactory. Many dentists using this method have fabricated their own bite-blocks from wood, plastic, or metal.

The bite-block method has two main advantages: (1) the patient does
Text continued on page 76

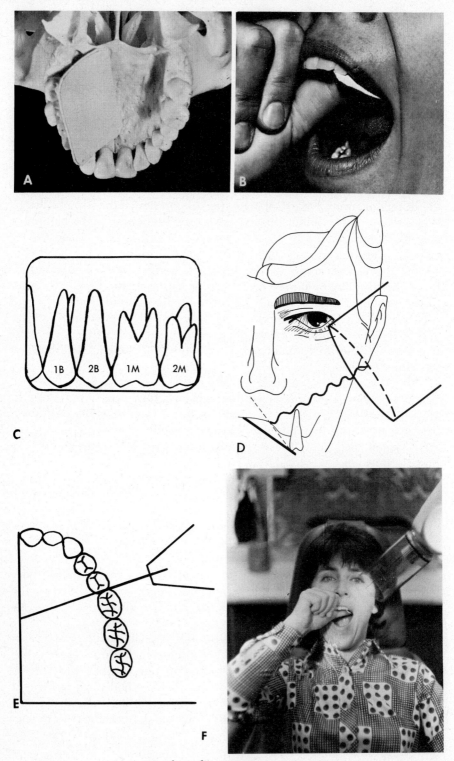

See legend on opposite page

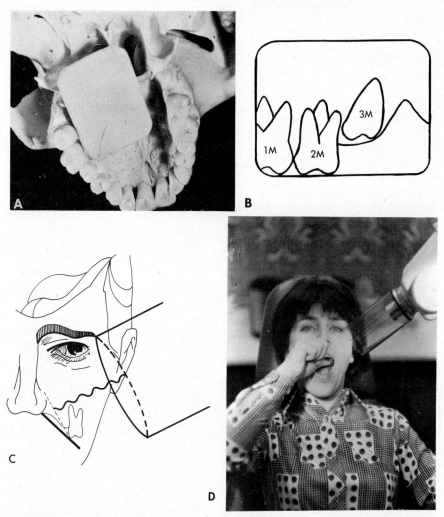

Figure 5–8   Maxillary molar exposure. *A,* Position of film over teeth on skull. *B,* Diagram of the teeth in relation to the film. *C,* Vertical angulation. *D,* Position of patient, film, and cone tip for exposure.

Figure 5–7   Bicuspid exposure. *A,* Position of film over teeth on skull. *B,* Patient holding film in position. *C,* Diagram of the teeth in relation to the film. *D,* Vertical angulation. *E,* Horizontal angulation. *F,* Position of patient, film, and cone tip for exposure.

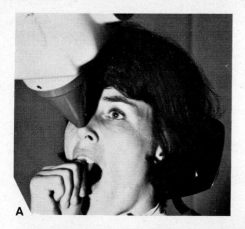

A

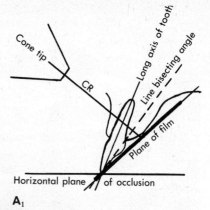

Cone tip

CR

Long axis of tooth

Line bisecting angle

Plane of film

Horizontal plane of occlusion

A₁

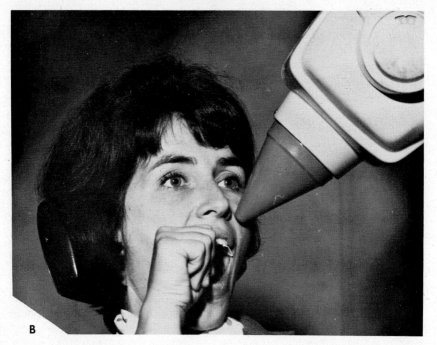

B

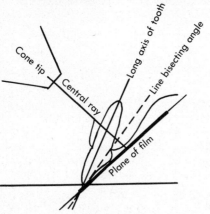

Cone tip

Central ray

Long axis of tooth

Line bisecting angle

Plane of film

B₁

Figure 5–9 Film, patient, and cone tip positioning when using the pointed plastic cone. *A* and *A₁*, Maxillary central and lateral exposure. *B* and *B₁*, Maxillary cuspid exposure.

Illustration continued on opposite page

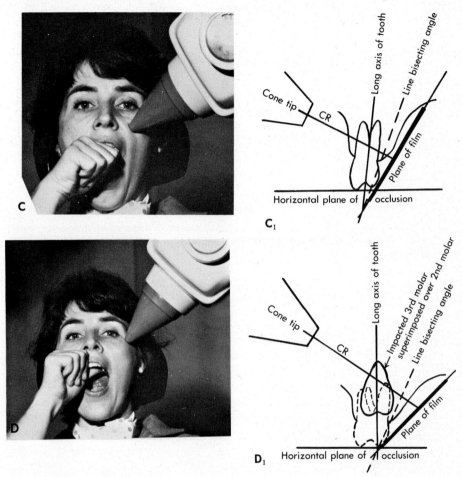

Figure 5–9 *Continued*   C and C_1, Maxillary bicuspid exposure. D and D_1, Maxillary molar exposure.

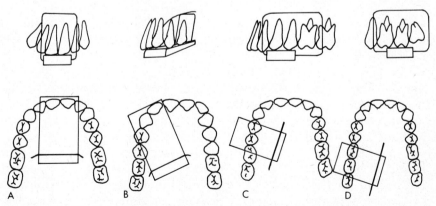

Figure 5–10   Use of the bite-block in the maxillary arch. *A*, Central and lateral incisor exposure. *B*, Cuspid exposure. *C*, Bicuspid-molar exposure. *D*, Third molar exposure.

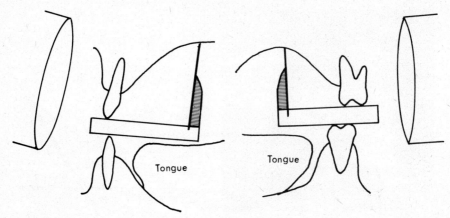

Figure 5–11   *A,* Film is placed deep in the palate for exposures of anterior teeth. *B,* Superior edge of the film is placed at the midline of the palate for the exposures of the posterior teeth.

not need to hold the film in position, and consequently his hand and fingers do not get exposed to repeated doses of primary radiation; (2) once the patient occludes on the bite-block, there is less chance for the film to move during the exposure. If there is a disadvantage it would be that with some patients the bite-block is difficult to position accurately, owing to an anatomical restriction. This increases the degree of discomfort to the patient when he occludes on the bite-block.

To acquaint yourself with the use of bite-blocks, see Figure 5–10, a series of diagrams showing a bite-block retaining the film in position. The procedure is as follows. Soften the corners of the film that will contact tissue; then place the film in the film holder. After positioning the film according to the diagrams, have the patient occlude firmly on the bite-block. Notice that the angle formed by the tooth and film is smaller than the angle formed when the digital retention method is used. The result is that less vertical angulation is used in most areas (Fig. 5–11). Again, it is a matter of just "bisecting the angle." Horizontal angulations are the same as those used for digital retention, except for the maxillary cuspid.

For the cuspid exposure the film is placed deeper in the palate. To pull the film closer to the cuspid would cause it to bend, increasing image distortion as well as patient discomfort. Because the film is positioned at a distance, the horizontal angulation is changed. The central ray must be directed through the labial surface of the cuspid on a line with the film. To project the central ray through the distal contact (60 degrees or more) would cause the shadow of the cuspid to be projected off the film. Overlap of cuspid and first bicuspid crowns cannot be avoided. Though unsatisfactory, it does not interfere with the periapical diagnosis.

REMINDERS

1. If the film is not positioned correctly, do not take the exposure.
2. After exposing the maxillary centrals at 0 degrees horizontal angulation, swing the tube head around to 60 degrees horizontal angulation when exposing the maxillary cuspid. This will provide you with a clearer exposure of the cuspid area.
3. When placing the film for a bicuspid, check to see if some fractional part of the cuspid is covered by the anterior edge of the film. This will ensure complete film coverage of the first bicuspid.
4. When placing the film for the maxillary third molar exposure, DO NOT LET THE PATIENT DICTATE TO YOU WHERE TO PLACE THE FILM. If a patient complains that the film is being placed back too far, explain to him why it must be placed correctly and use a topical spray to relieve the discomfort or gagging.
5. If your unit has an open-end short cone, the x-ray beam is more restricted in size than that with a pointed cone. You must visualize an extension of the cone going through the patient to the film. Is the film within the confines of the cone outline? If it isn't, chances are good that some part of the film will not be exposed (cone cutting).
6. Do not rely on the preset vertical angulations, which have been provided only as a guide in cone tip placement. Adherence to the bisection of the angle procedure is the only sure way of getting the best results.

6

EXPOSING PERIAPICAL FILMS OF THE MANDIBULAR ARCH

We judge ourselves by what we feel capable of doing, while others judge us by what we have already done.

Longfellow

The seven periapical films of the mandibular arch needed to make the full series of radiographs are the same as those of the maxillary arch; that is, the central and lateral incisor exposure, and both right and left exposures of the cuspid, bicuspid-molar, and third molar areas.

THE CENTRAL AND LATERAL INCISOR EXPOSURE (Fig. 6–1)

A. With the patient's mouth open, make the mandibular arch parallel to the floor by adjusting the headrest.

B. Place the film vertically in the patient's mouth, centering it over the contact point between the two central incisors.

C. The upper edge of the film should be parallel to and extend approximately 1/8 inch above the edges of the teeth.

D. Instruct the patient to hold the film in this exact position with either index finger. Check again to see that the mandibular arch is parallel to the floor.

E. Bisect the angle to establish the correct vertical angulation (approximately −30 degrees).

F. The horizontal angulation is established by directing the central rays through the midline of the patient's face.

G. Always point the central ray to the center of the film.

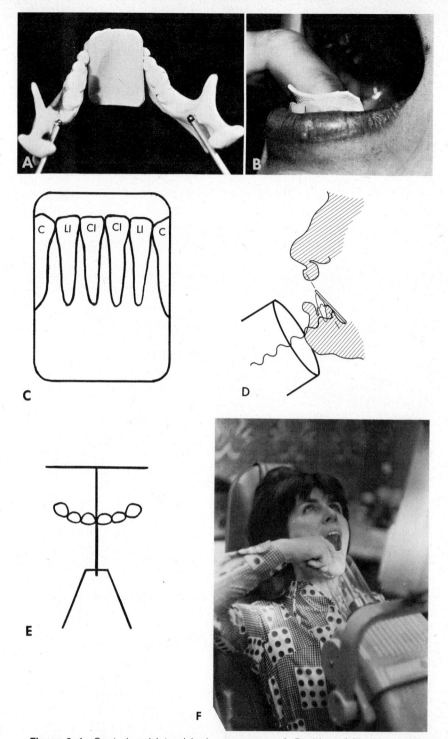

Figure 6–1 Central and lateral incisor exposure. *A,* Position of film over teeth on mandible. *B,* Patient holding film in position. *C,* Diagram of the teeth in relation to the film. *D,* Vertical angulation. *E,* Horizontal angulation. *F,* Position of patient, film, and cone tip for exposure.

THE CUSPID EXPOSURE (Fig. 6–2)

A. With the patient's mouth open, make the mandibular arch parallel to the floor.

B. Place the film vertically in the patient's mouth, centering it over the cuspid.

C. The upper edge of the film should be parallel to the occlusal line of the teeth and should extend approximately ⅛ inch above the incisal edge of the cuspid.

D. Instruct the patient to hold the film in this exact position, with the index finger opposite the side on which the film is placed. Check again to see that the mandibular arch is parallel to the floor.

E. Bisect the angle to establish the correct vertical angulation (approximately −30 degrees).

F. The horizontal angulation is established by directing the central rays through the contact point between the cuspid and first bicuspid.

G. Always point the central ray to the center of the film.

THE BICUSPID-MOLAR EXPOSURE (Fig. 6–3)

A. With the patient's mouth open, make the mandibular arch parallel to the floor.

B. Place the film horizontally in the patient's mouth, centering it over the contact point between the first molar and second bicuspid.

C. The upper edge of the film should be parallel to and extend ⅛ inch above the occlusal line of the bicuspid and molar teeth.

D. Instruct the patient to hold the film in this exact position, with the index finger opposite the side on which the film is placed. Check again to see that the mandibular arch is parallel to the floor.

E. Bisect the angle to establish the correct vertical angulation (approximately −15 to −20 degrees).

F. The horizontal angulation is established by directing the central rays parallel to the proximal surfaces of the bicuspid and molar teeth.

G. Always point the central rays to the center of the film.

THE THIRD MOLAR EXPOSURE (Fig. 6–4)

A. With the patient's mouth open, make the mandibular arch parallel to the floor.

B. Place the film horizontally in the patient's mouth, centering it over the third molar. (If the tooth is impacted, center the film over the third molar region.)

C. The upper edge of the film should be parallel to and even with the cusp tips of the first and second molars.

Text continued on page 86

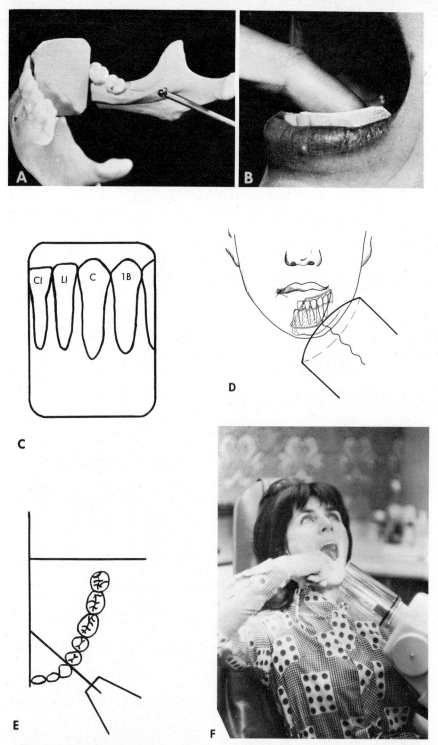

Figure 6–2 Cuspid exposure. *A*, Position of film over teeth on mandible. *B*, Patient holding film in position. *C*, Diagram of the teeth in relation to the film. *D*, Vertical angulation. *E*, Horizontal angulation. *F*, Position of patient, film, and cone tip for exposure.

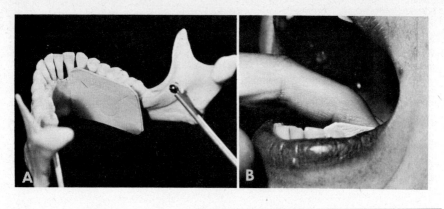

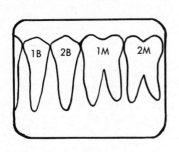

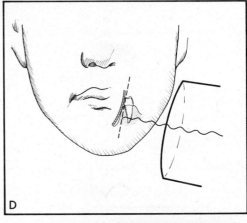

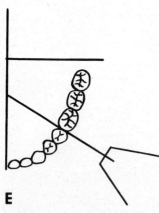

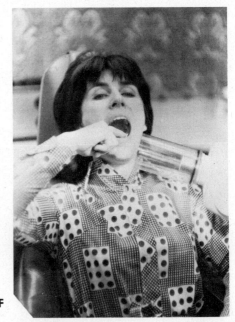

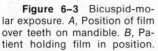

Figure 6–3 Bicuspid-molar exposure. *A*, Position of film over teeth on mandible. *B*, Patient holding film in position. *C*, Diagram of the teeth in relation to the film. *D*, Vertical angulation. *E*, Horizontal angulation. *F*, Position of patient, film, and cone tip for exposure.

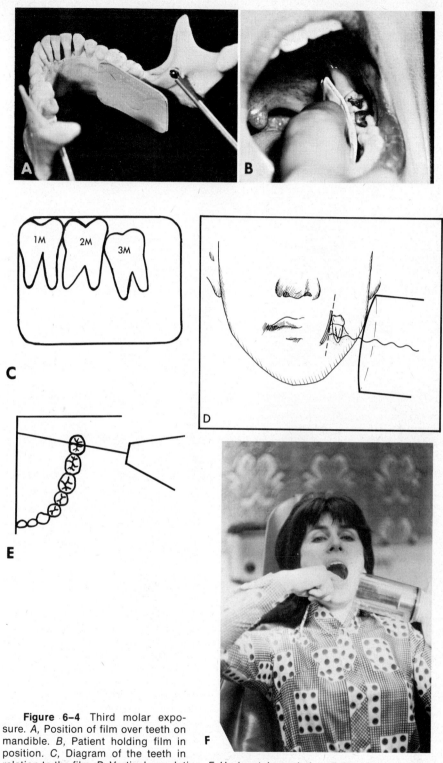

Figure 6–4 Third molar exposure. *A,* Position of film over teeth on mandible. *B,* Patient holding film in position. *C,* Diagram of the teeth in relation to the film. *D,* Vertical angulation. *E,* Horizontal angulation. *F,* Position of patient, film, and cone tip for exposure.

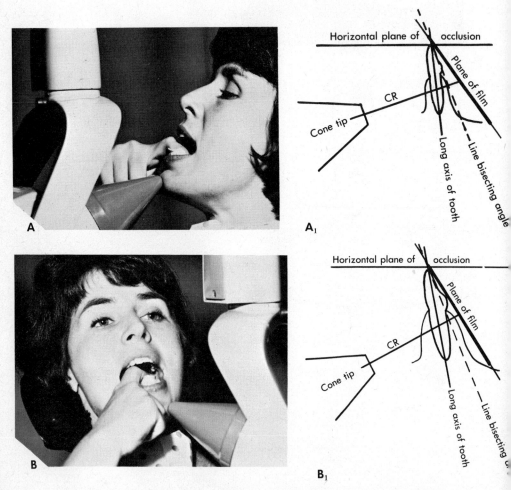

Figure 6–5 Film, patient, and cone tip positioning when using the pointed plastic cone. *A* and *A₁*, Mandibular centrals and laterals. *B* and *B₁*, Mandibular cuspids.

Illustration continued on opposite page

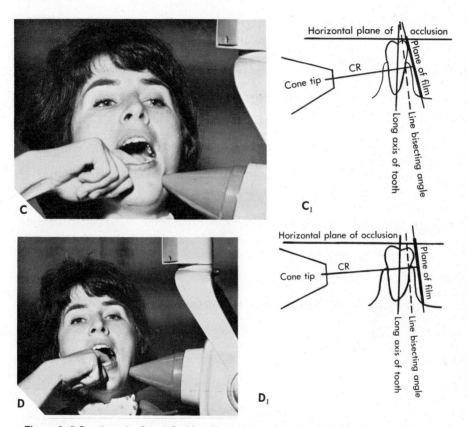

Figure 6–5 *Continued*   C and C_1, Mandibular bicuspids. D and D_1, Mandibular molars.

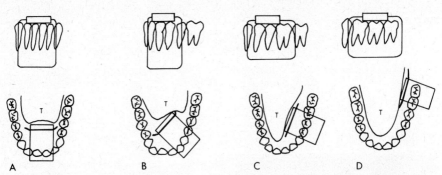

Figure 6–6 Use of the bite-block in the mandibular arch (T-tongue). *A*, Central and lateral incisor exposure. *B*, Cuspid exposure. *C*, Bicuspid exposure. *D*, Third molar exposure.

D. Instruct the patient to hold the film in this exact position, with the index finger opposite the side on which the film is placed.

E. Bisect the angle to establish the correct vertical angulation. In this region you will notice that the film lies parallel or nearly parallel to the tooth, owing to the flat surface of the mandible. Because of this parallelism there will be little or no vertical angulation (0 to −5 degrees).

F. The horizontal angulation is established by directing the central rays through the third molar region, parallel to the proximal surfaces of the molar teeth.

G. Always point the central ray to the center of the film.

Consult film manufacturer's instructions for dial settings and exposure time.

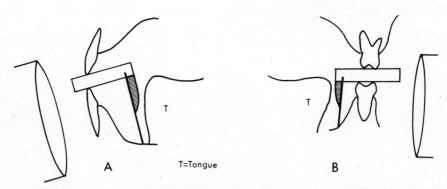

Figure 6–7 *A*, Film is moved slightly away from the anterior teeth. The tongue is easily displaced to make room for the film. *B*, Due to the shape of the mandible the film will be placed close to the bicuspid and molar teeth.

Film, patient, and cone tip positioning when using the pointed plastic cone for mandibular periapical exposures are shown in Figure 6–5.

THE BITE-BLOCK FILM HOLDER

As described in the preceding chapter, the use of a bite-block is an alternative to digital retention of the film. The diagrams in Figures 6–6 and 6–7 show correct positioning for the mandibular arch.

REMINDERS

1. After exposing the mandibular central incisors at 0 degrees horizontal angulation, swing the tube head around to 45 degrees horizontal angulation to expose the mandibular cuspid area. This will provide a clearer exposure of the cuspid area.
2. When placing the film for the mandibular centrals or cuspids, do not force it into the soft tissues. If you can't get the film down into the correct position, place it deep underneath the tongue at a greater angle. This will allow you to have the correct amount of film extending above the incisal edges.
3. Before placing the film for the lower bicuspids, soften the lower anterior corner to avoid cutting into the patient's tissues. If the mylohyoid muscle (which forms the floor of the mouth) is so tense that you have difficulty getting the film down to the prescribed position, use a bite-block film holder. When the patient closes on the bite-block, there is usually a relaxation of the mylohyoid muscle, allowing for correct placement of the film.
4. When placing the film for the mandibular bicuspids, the anterior edge of the film should cover some fractional part of the cuspid in order to ensure complete film coverage of the first bicuspid.
5. If you encounter a patient with a prominent lingual frenum (tissue leading from the tongue to the anterior alveolar ridge), it may be impossible to place the film satisfactorily for the central incisor exposure. Lay the film on top of the tongue and have the patient press on top of the film to hold it in position during the exposure. Since the angle formed by the teeth and film will be widened, you will need more minus vertical angulation to bisect the angle. (Owing to the interposed soft tissue of the tongue, the radiographic image will not have the clarity of a routine exposure.)

7

BITE-WING EXPOSURES

Everything yields to diligence.

Antiphanes

Bite-wing films should be included in a complete mouth survey of radiographs, because caries and the height of the alveolar crest are not seen with the greatest clarity in periapical exposures taken by means of the bisection of the angle technique. This is especially true in the bicuspid and molar regions. In the bite-wing technique the film is in a more parallel position with the teeth and supporting bone; for this reason we get better views of the areas affected by caries and of the condition of the supporting bone.

A posterior bite-wing on each side is usually all that is needed for children under 12. For adults, two posterior bite-wings on each side are recommended, because the curve of the arch may require two different horizontal angulations when moving from the bicuspid to the molar region. Some of the tooth surfaces can be seen on both bite-wing radiographs, which is advantageous because a questionable carious lesion can be verified on the second bite-wing radiograph. The two posterior bite-wings should be taken following the completion of the maxillary arch periapical films, because the maxillary arch must be parallel to the floor for both procedures. By including the bite-wings at this time, the patient's head will have to be adjusted only once more for the remaining mandibular films.

The regular No. 2 periapical film incorporated in a bite-wing tab is used for these exposures. The wing tab is placed on the stippled side of the film so that it divides the film in half horizontally for the posterior teeth and vertically for the anterior teeth. The upper half records the maxillary teeth and the lower half, the mandibular teeth. Carefully soften the corners of the film before inserting it in the mouth. This not only lessens the amount of time needed to place the film but also allows a more accurate film placement. Do not be concerned if the film appears to have a curved plane. Once in the mouth, the patient's tongue tends to straighten the film by exerting pressure against the teeth. Do be careful not to crease the film, as this will cause a dark streak through the radiograph. When placing the bite-wing film, make sure the film is equally divided between the maxillary and mandibular arches when the patient has closed on the tab. To do this, observe as the patient closes to see that the upper edge of the film is not caught by the cusps of the maxillary teeth, which would force the film downward over the mandibular teeth (Fig. 7–1).

BICUSPID BITE-WING EXPOSURE

A. Make the maxillary arch parallel to the floor.

B. For the patient's comfort, soften the anterior corners of the film by bending them away from the tab side of the film. Do not crease the film.

C. Center the lower half of the film over the contact point between the mandibular second bicuspid and the first molar (Fig. 7–2). (This will allow the cuspids to be observed on this film.) The bite-wing tab will lie over the occlusal surfaces of these teeth and is held temporarily in this position with your index finger (Fig. 7–3).

D. Instruct the patient to close slowly. The upper half of the film will bend to conform to the palate, a move facilitated by the softened corner of the film (Fig. 7–4). As the patient closes, roll your fingers to the buccal (outer) surfaces of the lower bicuspids, allowing the upper and lower teeth to occlude on the tab (Fig. 7–5). This will hold the film

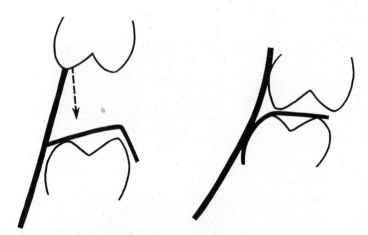

Figure 7–1 If film catches on upper cusp tips as patient closes, it will be forced down toward a periapical position with too much of the film extending below and not enough above.

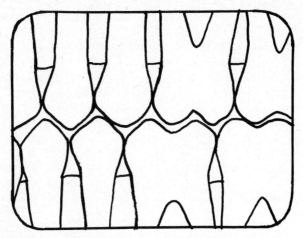

Figure 7-2 Diagram showing relation of teeth to film when the film is in position for the bicuspid bite-wing exposure.

in place during exposure. Be certain that the upper edge of the film has not engaged the cusps of the maxillary teeth. If this should occur, the film is forced downward out of correct position.

E. Center the cone over the bicuspids so that it points to the plane of occlusion. The vertical angulation is set at +10 degrees to offset the slight tilt of the upper half of the film (Fig. 7–6).

F. For the horizontal angulation, the central ray is directed through the interproximal space between the first and second bicuspids (as in the procedures for periapical exposures), approximately 70 to 80 degrees from the midline (Fig. 7–7).

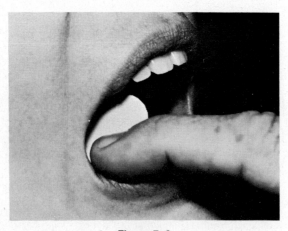

Figure 7-3

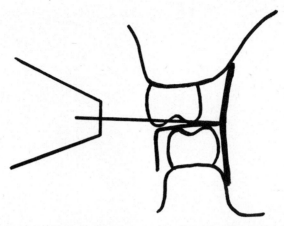

Figure 7–4   Diagram showing conformity of the film to the palate.

MOLAR BITE-WING EXPOSURE

For the molar bite-wing exposure, follow the same procedure as for the bicuspid bite-wing, with two exceptions: (1) the film is centered over the second molar (Fig. 7–8), and (2) the horizontal angulation of the cone is directed through the interproximal space between the first and second molar (Fig. 7–7). As with the bicuspid bite-wing exposure, the vertical angulation is +10 degrees (Fig. 7–9).

ANTERIOR BITE-WING EXPOSURE

When taking an anterior bite-wing exposure, the exceptions to this procedure are (1) the film is placed vertically and is centered over the

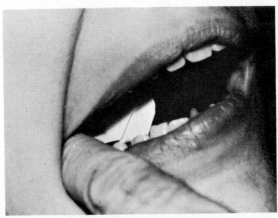

Figure 7–5

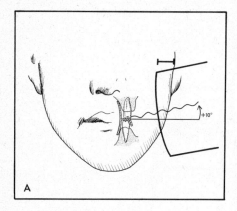

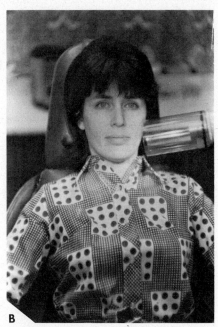

Figure 7–6 Position of patient, film, and cone for bicuspid bite-wing exposure.

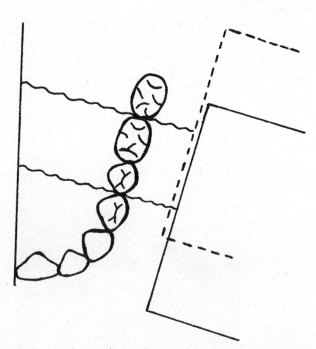

Figure 7–7 Horizontal angulation for bite-wing exposures. *Solid line* = bicuspid bite-wing. *Dotted line* = molar bite-wing.

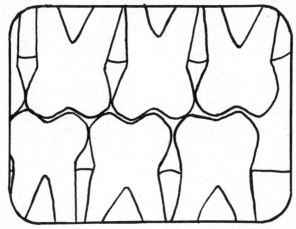

Figure 7–8   Diagram showing relation of teeth to film when the film is in position for the molar bite-wing exposure.

central incisors, the patient closing on the tab with the anterior teeth at an end-to-end occlusal relationship (Fig. 7–10); and (2) the central ray is directed through the midline.

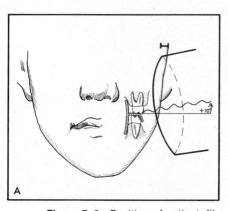
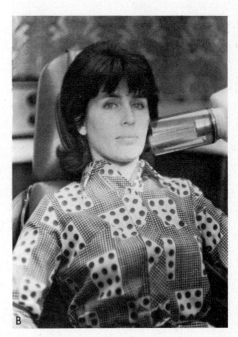

Figure 7–9   Position of patient, film, and cone for molar bite-wing exposure.

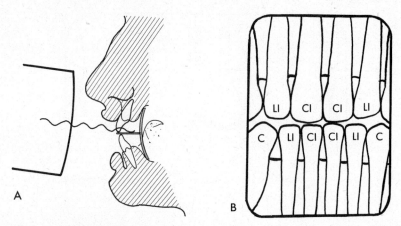

Figure 7–10 Diagrams showing relation of teeth to film when the film is in position for the anterior bite-wing exposure.

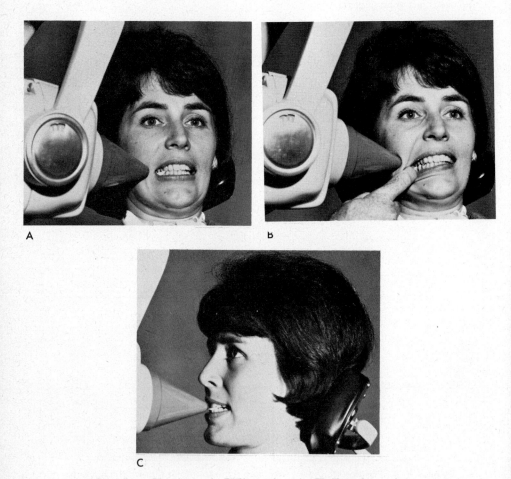

Figure 7–11 Position of patient, film, and cone tip when using the pointed cone. *A,* Bicuspid bite-wing. *B,* Molar bite-wing. *C,* Anterior bite-wing exposure.

In certain patients stabilization of the bite-wing tab may be difficult. Two examples follow.

Consider a patient whose lower molars are missing. To stabilize the bite-wing tab, place a cotton roll or folded gauze in the area of the missing teeth. When the patient closes, the upper molars will occlude against the gauze, thus supporting the tab. This situation arises with patients who wear partial dentures or removable bridges. Always remove these appliances, for failure to do so will superimpose the appliance over the teeth and ridge to which they are anchored.

Consider a patient with an edentulous (all teeth removed) upper arch, but with most or all of his lower natural teeth intact. If he is wearing an artificial denture in the upper arch, it may be kept in place for the exposure in order to stabilize the tab. If the patient is not wearing an upper denture, use gauze in place of the upper teeth to help stabilize the tab.

When using the pointed cone, the film placements and angulations are exactly the same as those used with the open-end short cone (Fig. 7–11).

REMINDERS

1. For patient comfort, always soften the corners of the film before placing it in the mouth, even though this will tend to bend the film. The tongue will flatten the film, reducing image distortion to a minimum.
2. The film must be equally divided between the maxillary and mandibular arches when the patient has closed on the tab.
3. The patient must occlude firmly on the bite-wing tab during the exposure.
4. The horizontal angulation used for the bite-wings is the same as that used for the periapicals of the same teeth.
5. The bicuspid and molar bite-wings have the same horizontal and vertical angulations.
6. The vertical angulation for bite-wing exposures is +10 degrees to the horizontal plane. The cone tip points DOWN at 10 degrees.

8

THE LONG CONE OR PARALLELING TECHNIQUE

Always behave like a duck—keep calm and
unruffled on the surface but paddle like the
devil underneath.

Jacob Braude

The long cone or "paralleling" technique, an alternate to the bisection of the angle technique, is preferred by many dentists. It produces the most accurate image of the teeth because it follows more of the principles of accurate shadow casting. The conditions which must be fulfilled to cast a shadow of an object as accurately as possible, as applied to radiographs of the teeth, are (1) the tooth must be parallel to and as close to the film as possible, and (2) the source of the x-rays must be small and as far from the tooth as possible.

The two obvious differences between the long cone and the bisection of the angle techniques are film placement and the distance from the target of the x-ray tube to the film (target-film distance).

The term paralleling technique indicates the manner in which the film is placed, i.e., parallel to the long axis of the tooth in question. In order to do this, the film must be positioned at a greater distance from the tooth to escape the restrictions of the oral anatomy. The first condition for accurate shadow casting is therefore only partly fulfilled, and the film is in closer proximity to the tooth in the bisection of the angle technique.

An intraoral film holder is necessary for this correct parallel placement (Fig. 8–1). It is a device usually made of plastic, wood, or metal which holds a periapical film far enough from the teeth and surrounding tissues to keep it parallel with the teeth to be exposed (Fig. 8–2). Some types of holders are held in position by biting upon them, and others by being held with the patient's fingers. Patients with low palates usually provide the most resistance to such film placement because

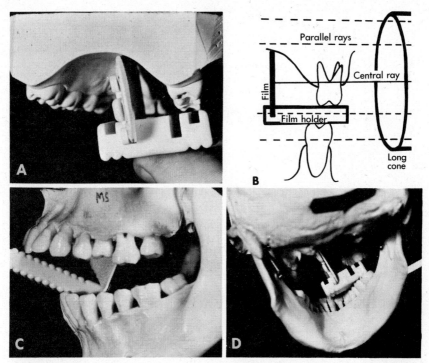

Figure 8–1 *A*, The film holder (Rinn XCP) allows the film to be placed at the center of the palate. *B*, A film holder being held in position by having the patient bite on it. *C*, For an exposure of the maxillary incisors the film is placed well back on the palate in order to maintain parallelism of the teeth and film. *D*, For exposing the maxillary posterior teeth the film should be placed at the midline of the palate.

the film tends to bend when it contacts the palate. The film should remain rigid and flat during the exposure, and the film support on the holder helps to maintain it in this position.

The target-film distance is increased 8 to 12 inches or more than the 8 inch length of the short cone. The long cone is a tubelike structure at least twice the length of the short cone and is merely a means by which we can accurately position the tube head from this greater distance (Fig. 8–3). Attempts to direct the central rays to the film without such a guide would be a difficult procedure. Another of the conditions for accurate shadow casting is fulfilled by this increased target-film distance because the central rays are more parallel to each other when they reach the film, thus reducing the degree of shadow magnification.

The lead diaphragm in the cone is small enough to let only the most central parallel rays through to radiograph the teeth, the remainder of the peripheral rays being absorbed by the lead.

The central ray is directed perpendicular to both the film and the teeth because they are parallel to one another. If you notice, after film placement, that a slight angle is formed by the teeth and film, a satisfac-

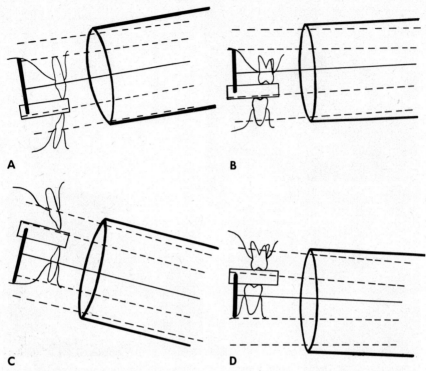

A

B

C

D

Figure 8–2 Position of the long cone in relation to the teeth and film. *A*, Maxillary anterior exposure. *B*, Maxillary posterior exposure. *C*, Mandibular anterior exposure. *D*, Mandibular posterior exposure.

tory shadow will be cast by directing the central ray perpendicular to the teeth. However, if the angle is greater than 15 degrees you should direct the ray according to the bisection of the angle technique. Failure to do so results in an elongated image. There will be patients in which it will be difficult or even impossible to come close to paralleling the film with the teeth and still have the patient occlude on the bite-block. In this case, remove the film from the bite-block, have the patient hold the film in the mouth with his finger, and then bisect the angle. There is still the advantage of the more parallel rays provided by the extended cone.

The intensity of radiation reaching the film is much less when the tube is moved back to the longer distance required in the long cone technique. An adjustment in the unit must be made to compensate for the greater target-film distance. The adjustments may be (1) increasing the kilovoltage peak, (2) increasing the milliamperage, (3) increasing the length of the exposure time, (4) increasing the speed of the film, or (5) any combination of the above. Assuming that the fastest speed film is being used, increasing the exposure time seems to be the most frequent change when making the transition from the short to the long cone.

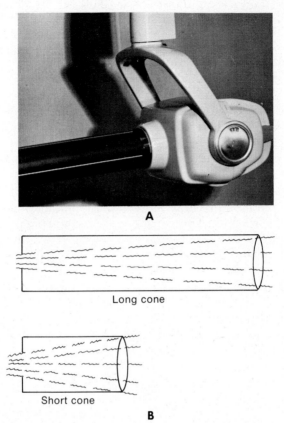

Figure 8-3 *A*, The tube head with a long cone attached to it. *B*, A sketch demonstrating the more parallel rays of the long cone in comparison with the more divergent rays of the short cone. (*A*, courtesy of the Ritter Equipment Co., Inc.)

The procedure for taking a full series of radiographs is the same as that described in Chapters 5, 6, and 7 for taking periapical and bitewing films. Horizontal film placement is the same, i.e., the film is centered over the same teeth for each exposure as in the bisection of the angle technique. One exception is that a No. 1 narrow periapical film may be used for the anterior region because it is more adaptable to this region of each arch. In this case a separate film of the lateral incisor is exposed in addition to the central incisor and cuspid exposures. The regular No. 2 periapical film is used for the remaining bicuspid and molar exposures.

FILM PLACEMENT

When employing the paralleling technique you will use two basic steps: (1) positioning the film as ideally as possible, and (2) positioning the cone correctly. There is no problem in positioning the cone, especially with today's sophisticated instruments that guide the cone into position. Therefore, if you can position the film satisfactorily, you will essentially have mastered the paralleling technique. The simplest and best way to place the film is by the "TPR" (Tilt-Position-Relax) method, described in the following paragraphs.

Tilt—For maxillary exposures tilt the film holder as you place it into the patient's mouth, trying not to contact any tissues until the film is in its proper position. The same procedure is used for mandibular exposures except for the posterior teeth when the cheek and tongue must be contacted during film placement. (See Fig. 8–4.)

Position—With the film still tilted, carefully position it exactly in line with the teeth you wish to radiograph, remembering that the central ray must be directed through the teeth to the center of the film. A common error is to upright the film into a vertical position as soon as it enters the mouth and then position it. This can be very irritating to the patient, especially when he tries to occlude on the bite-block.

Relax—As the patient begins to occlude on the bite-block, relax your grip on the bite-block handle. This will allow the film to move itself into the best possible placement for each patient. The patient must occlude firmly or the periapical areas of the teeth will not be adequately recorded on the resultant radiograph.

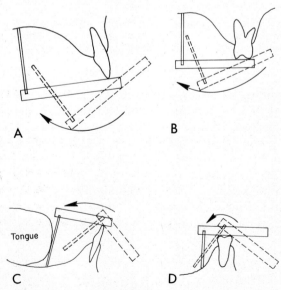

Figure 8–4 Dotted line demonstrates bite-block in tilted position as it enters the patient's mouth. Solid line demonstrates parallelism as the patient occludes on the bite-block. *A,* Maxillary anterior teeth. *B,* Maxillary posterior teeth. *C,* Mandibular anterior teeth. *D,* Mandibular posterior teeth.

Although the TPR formula may seem too simple to improve the results of this procedure, the proof will be in the quality of your radiographs. The following suggestions will further facilitate the placement of a film holder in the patient's mouth.

1. After you have positioned the film in the bite-block, always soften the corners of the film that contact soft tissue. This contributes greatly to patient comfort.

2. When exposing the maxillary anterior teeth, do not hesitate to place the film deep in the patient's mouth. This allows the film to parallel the teeth as much as possible. The patient will bite on the end of the bite-block if this procedure is followed correctly.

3. For exposures of the maxillary posterior teeth, place the bite-block in the mouth so that the superior edge of the film is at the midline or highest part of the palate. The patient will occlude on the end of the bite-block.

4. When placing the film for the lower anterior teeth, the film should parallel these teeth as much as possible. To achieve this, compress the tongue back in the mouth with the bite-block while placing the film in position. Having the patient close his mouth in a protrusive manner may aid you in this procedure.

5. There will be many instances in which your patient will have missing teeth, drifting teeth, and so forth. The bite-block may take an uneven position in the mouth when the patient closes his mouth. To maintain an even plane, place a cotton roll on the bite-block opposite the side the film is on. If you are exposing maxillary teeth, place the cotton roll between the mandibular teeth and the bite-block. For mandibular exposures, the roll is placed between the maxillary teeth and the bite-block. The cotton roll will fill the uneven areas of the occlusal plane, providing for a correct film position during the exposure.

EXTENSION CONE PARALLELING INSTRUMENTS (XCP)

Newer film holding instruments have been developed (Rinn-XCP) that have definite advantages over the regular bite-blocks. These instruments have an indicator rod with which the long cone is paralleled and a locator ring which allows you to direct the x-ray beam to the center of the film. There is an anterior instrument for radiographing the central-lateral incisor and the cuspid exposures and a posterior instrument for the posterior teeth exposures (Figs. 8–5, 8–6, and 8–7).

When using XCP instruments, lay the patient in a reclining position so that he is looking at the ceiling. By adjusting the patient's head slightly, all exposures may be made with the cone directed from overhead (Fig. 8–8).

These instruments may also be used with a unit having an open-end short cone; however, the image will not be as accurately produced

Text continued on page 110

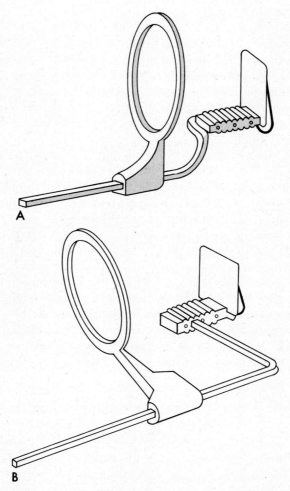

Figure 8–5 *A*, Anterior XCP instrument. *B*, Posterior XCP instrument.

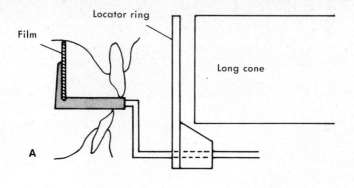

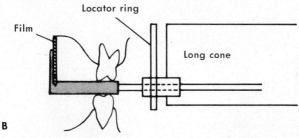

Figure 8–6 Film position using XCP instruments for (*A*) maxillary anterior teeth and (*B*) maxillary posterior teeth.

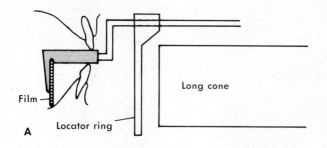

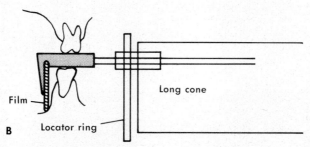

Figure 8–7 Film position using XCP instruments for (*A*) mandibular anterior teeth and (*B*) mandibular posterior teeth.

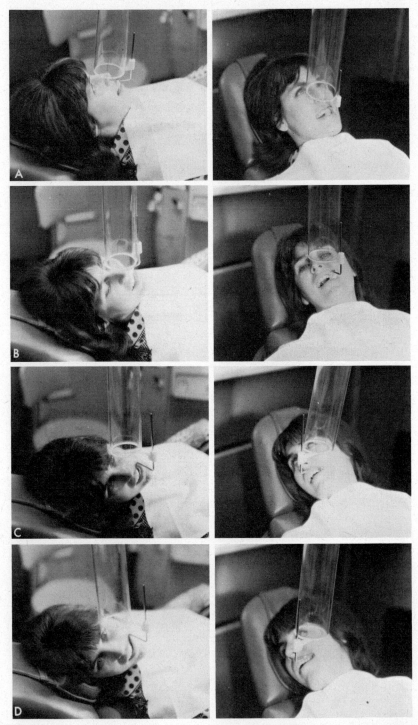

Figure 8–8   Position of patient, instrument, and extension cone (reclining position) for (A) maxillary central and lateral incisors, (B) maxillary cuspids, (C) maxillary bicuspids, (D) maxillary molars.

Illustration continued on opposite page

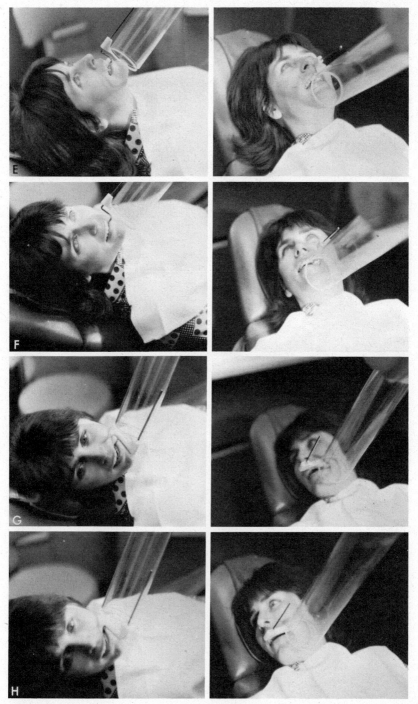

Figure 8–8 (continued)   (*E*) mandibular central and lateral incisors, (*F*) mandibular cuspids, (*G*) mandibular bicuspids, (*H*) mandibular molars.

Illustration continued on following page

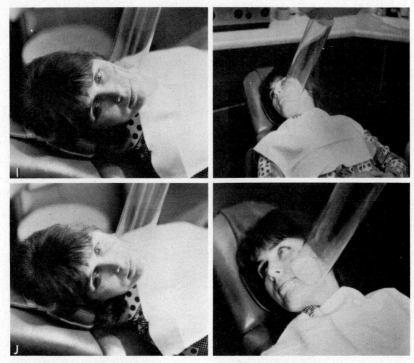

Figure 8–8 (continued)   (*I*) bicuspids bite-wing, and (*J*) molar bite-wing.

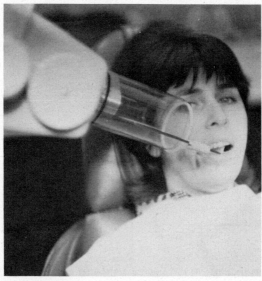

Figure 8–9   For all exposures, the position of patient, XCP instrument, and open-end short cone is the same as that used with the extension cone.

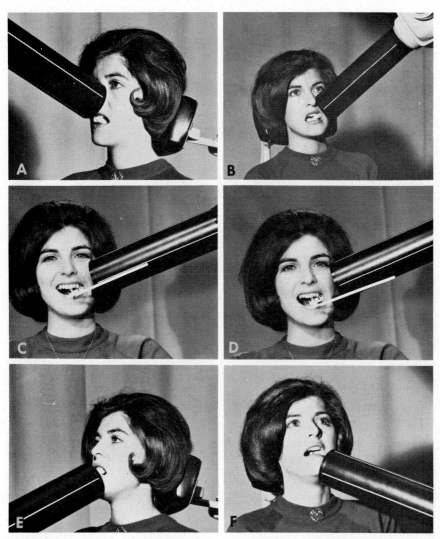

Figure 8–10 Relative positions of the long cone and the patient (upright position) for: *A*, Maxillary central incisor exposure. *B*, Maxillary cuspid exposure. *C*, Maxillary bicuspid-molar exposure. *D*, Maxillary third molar exposure. *E*, Mandibular central incisor exposure. *F*, Mandibular cuspid exposure.

Illustration continued on following page

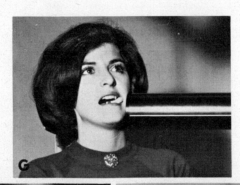

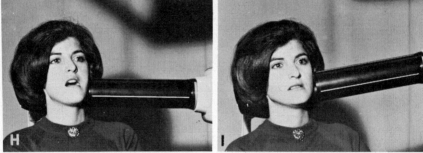

Figure 8–10 (continued) *G*, Mandibular bicuspid-molar exposure. *H*, Mandibular third molar exposure. *I*, Posterior bite-wing exposure using bite-wing tab.

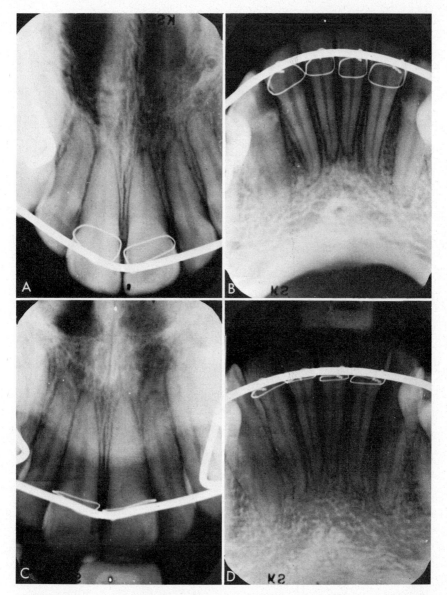

Figure 8–11   *A* and *B*, Radiographs of the maxillary and mandibular central incisor regions taken with a short cone using the bisection of the angle technique. *C* and *D*, Radiographs of the same region taken with a long cone using the paralleling technique. In both sets of radiographs the teeth are approximately the same length. However, in *C* and *D* the images of teeth and supporting bone are in a truer dimension. The labial and lingual orthodontic wires are superimposed over one another, which is the true relationship of these wires as they are placed in the mouth clinically. In *A* and *B* the wires appear circular. This result can be obtained only by exposing the radiographs at an angle many degrees from a line perpendicular to the teeth.

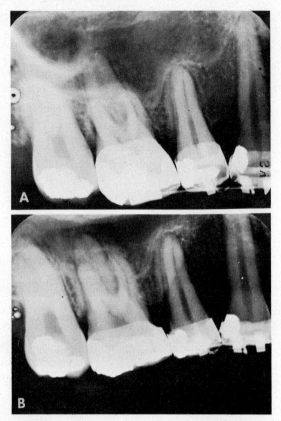

Figure 8–12   *A,* The maxillary bicuspid and molar teeth exposed using a short cone and the bisection of the angle technique. Because of the vertical angle at which it was exposed, the orthodontic bands appear to be higher on one side of the tooth than on the other. Also, the height of the alveolar bone crest is not in its true relation to the crown of the teeth. *B,* The same maxillary bicuspid and molar teeth exposed using the long cone and the paralleling technique. The orthodontic bands are projected in a much truer relationship, the buccal (outer) and lingual (inner) portions of the bands being superimposed over one another. The height of the alveolar bone is also correct in this radiograph.

as when the long cone is used. The short cone will tend to have some distortion as a result of the more divergent, somewhat conical x-ray beam. When using this setup, the parallel placement of film to teeth will produce a truer image than when the film is held by digital retention and the angle is bisected (Fig. 8–9).

Figure 8–10 shows the setups for the different areas when the long cone technique is used and the patient is in an upright position.

Figures 8–11 and 8–12 are radiographs of the same teeth comparing those taken by the bisection of the angle technique (short cone) to those taken with the paralleling technique (long cone). The degree of distortion you get with the bisection of the angle technique is obvious.

REMINDERS

1. Have someone place the film and the film holder in the different areas of your mouth so that you can experience what the patient feels.
2. To reduce discomfort to the patient, always soften the corners of the film that contact tissue.
3. Your number one goal is to PARALLEL the film with the tooth.
4. The patient MUST occlude on the bite-block during the exposure.
5. Bite-block instruments may be used in the same manner to record edentulous areas.
6. Patients will better tolerate discomfort in film placement if they know why the film must be placed up or down so far. When using this technique, keep in mind its mechanical superiority to the bisection of the angle technique.

9

REVIEW OF BASIC PRINCIPLES

All truly great ideas seem somewhat absurd when first proposed.

A. N. Whitehead

After many years of teaching I have noticed a number of common faults made by my students. The purpose of this chapter is to reemphasize the importance of following certain principles when radiographing your patients. What I want to do is to make the radiographic procedure as easy as possible for you, to help you produce the best possible radiographs, and to expose the patient to the least amount of radiation.

As you know, the two techniques for exposing intraoral radiographs are the bisection of the angle technique and the paralleling technique. The paralleling technique is the superior of the two for accuracy and image detail. However, the bisection of the angle technique definitely fulfills its purpose, for it also allows you to radiograph the periapical tissues with accuracy and reasonable image detail. In fact, most dentists use this technique. You should become competent in using the bisection of the angle technique first, then develop your skills for the paralleling technique. The reason for this is that there will be certain patients in whom the paralleling instruments cannot be placed accurately. You then have no choice but to use the bisection of the angle technique. Following are the basic principles you must follow to achieve your objectives when using the bisection of the angle technique.

BISECTION OF THE ANGLE TECHNIQUE

1. Position the Patient's Head Correctly
Adjust the headrest so that the arch being radiographed is parallel to the floor, the midsagittal plane perpendicular to the floor. This important rule is very seldom followed, especially by those just learning

112

this technique. It is a must if you wish to produce quality radiographs. Don't be satisfied with positioning the head "close enough"—position it EXACTLY as stated.

If you are observant you will notice that after you have positioned the patient's head correctly he often will alter this position each time you place a film in his mouth. This is an attempt on his part to help you. Do not discourage this effort, for it does make it easier for you to place the film. The important thing to remember is to CORRECTLY REPO-SITION THE PATIENT'S HEAD AFTER EACH FILM PLACE-MENT!

For example, after positioning the patient's head according to the rule, he may raise his head by forcing it against the headrest as you approach his mouth with the film. He is trying to help you. Fine! But don't leave the head in this incorrect position. After placing the film, put both of your hands on the sides of the patient's head and, using a gentle downward force, tell him to lower his head. Lower the head until the maxillary arch is parallel and the midsagittal plane is perpendicular to the floor.

If your radiographs tend to produce an elongated image of the maxillary teeth, double check to see that the patient's head is correctly positioned. Leaving the head in an upward tilt has the same effect as decreasing the vertical angulation of the x-ray beam. The result: elongated images of the teeth, especially the anterior teeth.

When bite-wing exposures are taken, the patient tends not only to raise his head up and back but also to tilt it to one side or the other. This is particularly true if you haven't softened the corners of the film, since it hurts when closing on the tab. As with periapical film placements, after the patient occludes on the bite-wing tab place one hand on each side of the face and position the head EXACTLY as prescribed. Again, *reposition the head after each film placement.*

2. Place the Film Correctly

The second basic rule concerns film placement and can be summed up in three words: *Do not compromise!* Never let the patient dictate where you will place the film in his mouth. If you have had any practical experience in taking radiographs, you know that there are patients who will complain about the entire x-ray procedure and possibly even become irate as you try to position the film. The two most unpopular placements are those for the maxillary molars and the mandibular bicuspids. The former causes the patient to gag and the latter hurts. Regardless of the complaints, the film must cover the area of interest or it will not show on the resultant radiograph.

For the maxillary molar placement, the film *must* be centered anteroposteriorly over the second molar, so as to record the third molar (if present) and the complete maxillary tuberosity. Even if the patient gags or complains that the film is placed too far back in his mouth you must not reposition it more comfortably at the expense of obtaining an inadequate radiograph. You may use a topical anesthetic spray or some other means to permit you to place the film where it belongs, but DO NOT COMPROMISE. It will do no good to place the film incorrectly to appease the patient. Radiographing the proper area is essential for a proper diagnosis.

For the mandibular teeth, the film must be down far enough to record the apex and surrounding bone. If the apex of each tooth, with its surrounding bone, is not recorded on the radiographs, then by definition the films taken are not "periapical," they are "half-root." Needless to say, these films are of poor diagnostic quality.

Retakes cost time and money, but the more serious problem is reexposure of the patient. This hazard can be eliminated by taking the right exposure the first time through convincing yourself that there is no room for compensatory measures when placing each film in its predetermined position.

3. Take a Complete Radiographic Series

A common error is the taking of an incomplete radiographic series. A series of radiographs is not complete unless exposures are taken of *all* areas, including those where there are two or more teeth missing. As an example, consider the case of a patient who has had three molars extracted in the mandibular molar area. This patient probably has a partial denture to make up for the loss of his natural teeth. Even though the tissues appear normal and healthy clinically, treat the area as if teeth were present and take the radiograph. Make no exceptions. Many innocent looking edentulous ridges have yielded underlying problems when examined radiographically. Failure to take the complete series may result in future legal problems. Enough said.

4. Take High-Quality Radiographs

Never be satisfied with radiographs unless they are of the highest quality. A poor series of radiographs will reflect not only on your ability but also on your attitude concerning the end results. If a retake or two (or three) is needed because of a technical error, proceed with the retake exposures but make sure you understand what you did wrong the first time and make the necessary corrections. No one likes retakes, but it is infinitely better than trying to guess what is or is not present on a radiograph of poor diagnostic quality. Lest you forget, should legal problems arise with a patient, radiographs are of prime importance in that they are factual evidence.

PARALLELING TECHNIQUE

The principles reviewed so far in this chapter apply to the paralleling technique as well as to the bisection of the angle technique. However, when using the paralleling technique the head position is not quite so critical. The film-holding instruments, and application of the simple "90 degrees to the long axis of the tooth" rule, make the setting of the vertical angulation easier to determine regardless of the patient's head position. You will also notice that the film-holding instruments have a ridged backing to support the film. At times this causes more discomfort to the patient than does the digital retention method, but keep the second basic principle in mind and do not compromise on film placement. Principles 3 and 4 are self-explanatory and are of equal importance for both techniques.

10

RECOGNIZING AND SOLVING PROBLEM SITUATIONS

It is never too late to be what you might have been.

George Eliot

Most textbooks on dental radiography provide excellent instructions for step-by-step radiographic procedures. Patients with "ideal" dental arches are used in the photographs so that you may see how the film should be placed, where the cone is positioned, and so on. However, taking radiographs of the "ideal" dental patient is an infrequent experience, for you will find that most patients present one or more problems. The purpose of this chapter is to help you to solve these problems by using variations in your x-ray techniques. The first section is devoted to the bisection of the angle technique; the second to the paralleling technique.

BISECTION OF THE ANGLE TECHNIQUE

Abnormal Arch Morphology

I. The Narrow "V"-Shaped Maxillary Arch

The narrow maxillary arch creates a problem primarily when placing films in the anterior segment, especially the cuspid areas. The difficulty is that there is not enough space to place the film high enough to record the apices of the teeth. For the maxillary cuspid, the anterosuperior corner of the film contacts the posterior teeth or palate on the opposite side, thereby preventing proper placement. Difficulty is also encountered during the bicuspid film placement. The film can't be placed high enough to record the apices or anteriorly enough to cover the cuspid and, in some cases, the first bicuspid. Film placement for the molar exposure is usually not affected by the narrow palate.

A. *Central Incisor Exposure*

Proceed in the same manner as you would if the palate were normal in width, centering the film over the contact point between the two central incisors. When using finger retention, the patient should not try to force the film into contact with the palate, as this will cause the film to bend too much through its short axis, producing severe image distortion, especially of the lateral incisors. Have the patient use light finger pressure which will still produce some bending but not enough to be objectionable. The coronal portion of the film may move away from the crowns of the teeth, but this will not be significant enough to cause any major image distortion (Fig. 10–1).

The alternative would be to lay the film in a flat plane over the incisal edges and cusp tips of the teeth. However, this method of placement has its drawbacks. There is a greater chance of vertical distortion owing to the greater angle to bisect, and the increased distance between the tooth apex and the film will cause lack of clarity in the apical region. With either type of film placement, always do your best to accurately bisect the angle.

B. *Cuspid Exposure*

When taking x-rays of the maxillary cuspid of a narrow palate, it is nearly impossible to place the film up on the palate as you normally do without severe film bending (Fig. 10–2). To make the best of a poor situation, "cross-arching" is the only practical method of film placement (see Cuspid Exposure, Chapter 5). The film is centered over the cuspid to be radiographed with the apical end of the film placed against the occlusal surfaces of the teeth on the opposite side of the maxillary arch. Very light finger pressure should be used to retain the film in position. Bowing of the film between the two arches from excessive pressure must be prevented, as this will cause a distorted image.

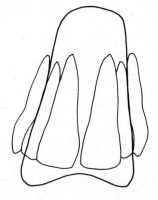

Figure 10–1 Maxillary central incisor film placement for a patient with a narrow "V"-shaped maxillary arch. Some bending through the short axis of the film is permissible.

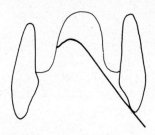

Figure 10-2 Excessive bending through long axis of film will produce image distortion.

Horizontal Angulation. The horizontal angulation for both the above exposures is the same as that used for the normal patient. The central ray is directed through the midsagittal plane (0 degrees) for the maxillary central exposure and through the contact point between the cuspid and bicuspid (approximately 60 to 70 degrees from the midsagittal plane) for the cuspid exposure.

C. Bicuspid Exposure

You will usually experience difficulty in placing the film anteriorly over the cuspid (in some cases, the first bicuspid) owing to the anatomical restrictions of the palate. Forcing the film up into the midline of the palate will cause severe film bending and may be quite irritating to the patient (Fig. 10-3). Also you may find that too much of the film extends below the occlusal plane when you try to position it in a routine manner.

The most successful method of film placement is as follows. Carry the film into the mouth in a flat plane parallel to the floor (0 degrees horizontal). With the anterior edge of the film in line with the cuspid, lay the film gently into contact with the opposite side of the palate. Have the patient use very light finger pressure to retain the film in position without bowing or bending. Remember that the film must be in the mouth deep enough to record the apical areas of the teeth. The horizontal angulation is determined by directing the central ray through the open contact point between the two bicuspids, usually at an angle of 65 to 70 degrees from the midsagittal plane.

With the above three exposures the film lies in a more horizontal

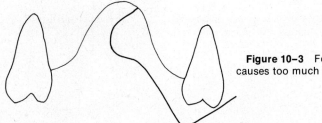

Figure 10-3 Forcing film into position causes too much film bending.

plane than that routinely seen. In essence, this increases the angle between the film and the tooth. When bisecting the angle you will direct the vertical setting of the tube head higher than you would for the average patient.

D. Molar Exposure

The molar film position does not usually pose a problem. Proceed in the usual manner.

E. Bite-Wing Exposure

When exposing the bicuspid bite-wing radiographs you can expect difficulty in placing the film anteriorly enough to include the cuspids. In this case you must roll and soften the corners of the film. Keep the bite-wing tab flat and allow the film to move away from the teeth. This will position the superior film edge more toward the highest part of the palate, decreasing the overall bending of the film. With the film softened and allowed to drift away from the teeth, the patient should have little trouble in occluding on the edge of the film tab (Fig. 10–4).

For the molar bite-wing exposure, the palate is usually high enough for an adequate film placement. The problem area is more often the prominent alveolar process on the lingual side of the maxillary arch. To counteract the film bending that would be caused by this bony prominence, again allow the film to move toward the tongue as the patient closes. The patient will bite on the end of the tab in the same manner as for the bicuspid bite-wing (Fig. 10–5).

Vertical Angulation.   The vertical angulation for both exposures will be the same as that used for any other bite-wing: +10. If the patient has a pronounced V-shaped arch, the horizontal angulation will be more toward 60 to 65 degrees from the midsagittal plane.

II. The Narrow Mandibular Arch

It would follow that if the maxillary arch is narrow, the mandibular arch would have to conform to the narrow contour if the teeth are going to occlude properly. Here again the placement of film for the centrals and cuspids will be the most difficult of the lower arch.

As an aid to placing the film in the first two exposures (central incisor and cuspid) it is suggested that you use the "anterior grasp" tech-

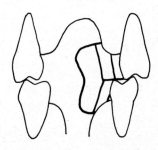

Figure 10–4 Softening the corners of the film allows a more accurate film placement for the bicuspid bite-wing.

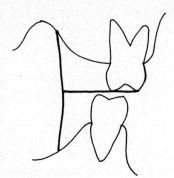

Figure 10–5 Allowing the film to move a short distance from the posterior teeth will result in greater image clarity.

nique. As you can see in Figure 10–6, the film is curved through its short axis; this is the same curvature it will assume in the mouth when it is positioned. Place the film on top of the thumb and third finger. The index finger presses on top of the film, forcing it to bend through its short axis. This bending does not cause any discernible distortion of the film image. On the contrary, the anterior grasp discourages bending through the long axis of the film, which does produce severe distortion. As you position the film, do not force it directly down into the soft tissue in an attempt to keep it close to the teeth. Rather, place it at an angle and carry it deep underneath the tongue. This will facilitate its placement to the correct depth and is much less irritating to the patient (Fig. 10–7A and B). As the patient applies just enough finger pressure to retain the film in position, the film will move somewhat closer to the teeth, thereby allowing you to project a more accurate shadow on the radiograph. You then apply the bisection of the angle principle to complete the exposure.

A. *Central Incisor Exposure*

Using the anterior grasp, place the film deep underneath the tongue to record the apical areas. There is usually not enough room to position the film in a more upright manner. As the patient retains the

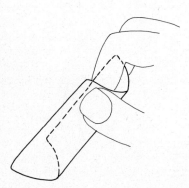

Figure 10–6 The "anterior grasp" for film placement of the mandibular anterior teeth.

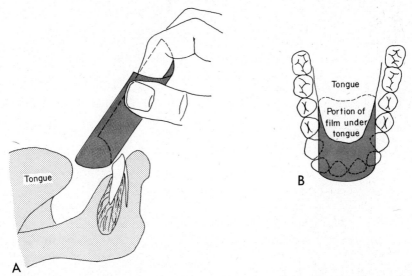

Figure 10–7   *A,* Placing the film at an angle to the teeth. *B,* Film placed at an angle deep under the tongue.

film in position with finger pressure, there will be considerable bending through the short axis of the film. The cuspids will appear distorted as a result of the extreme curvature of the film, but under these conditions the distortion is not objectionable. Another method would be to use a film holder and position the film with some degree of parallelism to the central incisors. The distance between the right and left bicuspids is usually less than the width of the film, which may prevent you from placing the film down far enough to record the apical regions. However, there is no harm in trying.

  B. Cuspid Exposure

  For this exposure, first try to place the film as you normally would. If your placement isn't close enough to what it should be, you have two alternatives:

  1. Position the film exactly as you would for the central incisor exposure, but direct the x-ray beam through the cuspid at a horizontal angulation of 45 degrees to the midsagittal plane. There is then enough of the film covering the cuspid to get an accurate image of the cuspid itself, all other structures being blurred out. Be sure to bisect the angle, as there is a tendency toward not using enough vertical angulation (Fig. 10–8).

  2. The other method is the "cross-arch" film placement. Center the film over the cuspid to be radiographed. The inferior edge of the film, instead of being placed deep underneath the tongue, will lie over the occlusal surfaces of the posterior teeth on the opposite side of the arch.

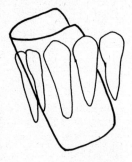

Figure 10–8 Film placement for the mandibular central incisors of the "V"-shaped arch may be used when exposing the cuspid.

The film plane may be kept flat, with the patient using very light finger pressure to retain the film in position. Bisect the angle.

C. Bicuspid and Molar Exposures

Other than a tense mylohyoid muscle creating a shallow sulcus, the narrow mandibular arch does not cause problems of any significance in these areas.

Normal Arch Morphology

I. Maxillary Arch

Most patients will not have exceptionally narrow dental arches nor will they have large tori (enlarged protuberances of bone) to interfere with proper film placement. Except for an occasional malpositioned tooth, most patients have palates of normal width and height. However, there are two areas that may present some degree of difficulty when trying to place a film accurately.

A. Cuspid Exposure

You may not be able to place the film high enough on the palate to accurately record the apex of the cuspid. The anterosuperior corner of the film contacts the bicuspid area of the opposite side of the palate, leaving an excess amount of film protruding below the cusp tip of the cuspid. If the film is left in this position, the periapical area of the cuspid will be omitted from the resultant radiograph. In order to record the apical area you must rotate the film anteriorly. The superior corner that made the premature contact with the opposite bicuspid will slide posteriorly. With this new "oblique" position, the cuspid will be viewed on the film in a corner-to-corner position rather than in the standard edge-to-edge. This positional change of the film is acceptable in light of the fact that the periapical area may now be viewed on the radiograph. Have the patient use just enough pressure to retain the film. Bending the film through its long axis must be avoided, as this will cause elongated images. When you position the cone, don't forget to direct the horizontal angulation through the contact point between the cuspid and the bicuspid. Horizontal overlap between these two teeth should be avoided (see Cuspid Exposure, Chapter 5).

B. Molar Exposure

Gagging. Not infrequently you will encounter patients who tend to gag at the slightest stimulation to the palate, especially in the molar area. Such patients may appear calm and stoic, but the truth is that they are actually quite nervous and fearful, which lowers the threshold to the gag reflex.

The first and probably the best counteractant to the gag reflex is a calm, reassuring voice. Through this type of communication the patient will rapidly develop confidence in you, which will allay his fear and apprehension proportionately. Of course it goes without saying that you never ask a patient, "Are you a gagger?" All this does is set the stage for the gag reflex. Do not even mention the subject.

Another very helpful step to prevent gagging is to place the film in a gentle, nonirritating manner. Carry the film back in air space, touching neither the tongue nor the palate. Once the film is adjacent to the maxillary tuberosity, lay it softly against the palatal tissues and the molar teeth. The patient retains the film with light finger pressure directed against the crown-gingival junction of the molar teeth.

If you still meet with resistance, some patients will respond favorably to the taste of salt on their tongue. (Check first to be sure that the patient is not on a salt-free diet.) Have the patient touch his tongue to some salt placed in the palm of his hand.

As a last resort, use a topical anesthetic spray or troche and always follow directions accordingly. These must be administered by the dentist.

II. Mandibular Arch

Problems with film placement seldom arise in a patient with a normal mandibular arch. The one problem that may occur is not being able to get the film down far enough to record the apices of the teeth. If you try to place the film straight up and down in a manner closely paralleling the long axis of the teeth, it may meet with resistance where the mylohyoid muscle attaches to the mandible.

Three steps may be used to obtain satisfactory results. First, use positive gentle communication to make the patient relax in general. A tense patient means a tense mylohyoid muscle. You can tell when the patient has relaxed, for the film placement becomes much easier.

Next, try to place the film at a greater angle to the tooth, allowing the inferior edge to be placed deep underneath the tongue. Only 1/8 to 1/4 of an inch of the film should extend above the occlusal plane. This is essential if the apical areas of the teeth are to be recorded.

The third step is one used with consistent success for all exposures of the mandibular arch: the use of a film holder. Film holders are routinely used with the paralleling technique, but they can also be used with the short cone for mandibular exposures. (In the maxillary arch the tooth-film distance, increased by the use of the film holder, would tend to produce an excess of image magnification.) As the patient closes on the film holder, the mylohyoid muscle tends to relax, especially in the bicuspid area. Patient discomfort can be reduced by softening the inferior corners of the film. Again, do not position the film straight up and down, but rather at an angle to the tooth. Relax your grip on the film holder as the patient occludes. This will allow minor movement of the film holder to better adapt the film to the patient's anatomical structures. There will be some degree of angulation between the tooth and the film (with the possible exception of the mandibular molar exposure), so you will still have to bisect the angle.

III. Variants of Normal Arches

A. Positional Differences of the Central and Lateral Incisors

The first variant is the patient with maxillary central incisors that are recessed and slanted lingually, with the lateral incisors overlapping labially (Fig. 10–9A). Since the central and lateral incisors are usually x-rayed with one film, the problem arises as to which angle to bisect—the angle formed by the central incisors and the film, or that formed by the lateral incisors and the film. If the angle bisected is formed by the centrals and the film, the laterals will probably appear elongated (Fig. 10–9B). If the angle bisected is formed by the laterals, the centrals will usually appear foreshortened, the severity of the distortion depending upon the angular differential between the central and the lateral as they are positioned in the arch (Fig. 10–9C). You have a choice. Take two exposures (bisecting each of the above angles) or bisect the angle formed by the laterals and the film, with the attitude of accepting foreshortened central incisors. At least the apical region of the centrals can be observed. If the angle formed by the centrals and the film is bisected, you risk having the lateral incisors so elongated

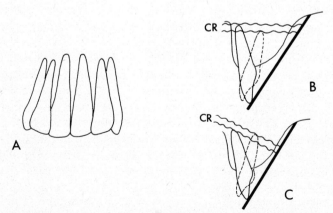

Figure 10–9 *A,* Recessed maxillary central incisors with overlapping lateral incisors. *B,* Bisecting the angle formed by the central incisors and the film. *C,* Bisecting the angle formed by the lateral incisors and the film.

that a satisfactory view of their apical regions may not be on the result-ant radiograph.

B. *Lingual Slant of Mandibular Anterior Teeth*

No doubt you have had patients with an exaggerated overbite. The lower anterior teeth most always tilt lingually. Though the film will be positioned in a normal manner, the bisecting plane assumes a more ver-tical direction. Therefore the central ray will be directed near a vertical angulation of 0 degrees when bisecting the angle. To guard against ex-cessive film bending, only enough finger pressure should be used to re-tain the film in position and NO MORE!

C. *Bite-wing Exposures of Ectopically Positioned Teeth*

Another common variant is the lingually positioned bicuspid (ei-ther arch). Though other teeth may be ectopically positioned, the bicus-pid is most often found displaced from an otherwise normal arch align-ment. In most cases it will be impossible to open either one or both contact points when exposing a "routine" bite-wing radiograph of this area.

The procedure to follow is to take a bite-wing exposure of this area to obtain a radiographic reading of the interproximal spaces of the nor-mally aligned teeth (Fig. 10–10A). Next, have the patient bite into a quarter-inch–thick pad of beeswax, forcing the wax into the interprox-imal areas of the displaced tooth. Remove the wax pad and observe the raised portions of the interproximal wax. This indicates the direction the central rays should travel to open the respective contacts on either side of the tooth. As you can see, it is possible that three bite-wing ex-posures of the same area may be necessary (Figs. 10–10B and C).

The procedure for exposing a periapical film of the displaced tooth does not usually pose a problem, because the long axis of the displaced tooth closely parallels the long axis of the other teeth. Though the film may be prevented from contacting the other teeth when positioning it, always bisect the angle formed by the film and the teeth in normal alignment.

D. *Overlapping Maxillary First and Second Molars*

The horizontal overlap of the interproximal surfaces is often seen between the maxillary first and second molars. Assuming your tech-nique is correct, you will find that all interproximal contacts will be open except in this area. Upon closer clinical examination you can see that the maxillary second molar has positioned itself around buccally to the first molar. This explains the resultant overlap, which may be cor-rected by taking a separate bite-wing exposure. Position the bite-wing film normally and direct the central ray at an angle of approximately 65 degrees to the midsagittal plane instead of 75 degrees (Fig. 10–11). The resultant radiograph should exhibit an open contact between the two molars. Don't be alarmed if all other contacts are overlapped—you have a clear view of these contacts on your original bite-wing radiograph. A

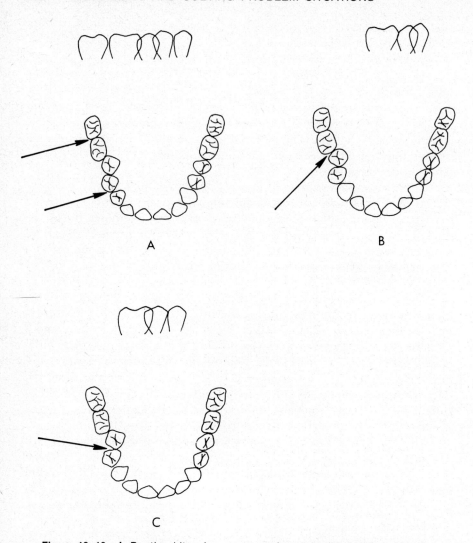

Figure 10–10 *A,* Routine bite-wing exposure demonstrating horizontal overlap of both interproximal surfaces of ectopically positioned tooth. *B,* Horizontal angulation used to open the distal contact point. *C,* Horizontal angulation used to open the mesial contact point.

beeswax impression of these teeth may also aid you in directing the cone for this additional exposure.

E. Maxillary and Mandibular Tori

These bony protuberances may cause difficulty, especially when you are positioning film for periapical exposures. The significance of this problem depends upon the size of the tori. "Large" tori are those tori whose size prevents normal film positioning. A large maxillary torus will not allow you to position the film high enough to record the molar apices. With certain procedural changes you may be able to ob-

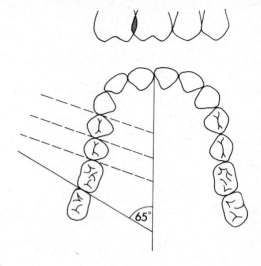

Figure 10–11 Horizontal angulation (approximately 65°) used to open contact point between the maxillary first and second molars. *Dotted lines =* routine 75° horizontal angulation. *Solid line =* horizontal angulation changed to 65°.

tain a radiograph that can be used as a diagnostic aid, but do not expect it to be as clear or sharp as a normal radiographic image. The reason is twofold: (a) the density of bone comprising the torus is greater than that of the surrounding bone and will usually be superimposed over the apical region of the molar teeth; (b) the film will be contacting the tori and the teeth instead of the palate and the teeth. This means that the apical half of the film lies still farther from the tooth apices, resulting in a greater penumbra of the root images.

For maxillary teeth, position the film so that no more than one quarter of an inch extends below the incisal edges or occlusal plane of the teeth. The apical end of the film will lie over the tori. The film has no support between the teeth and the tori; therefore, to prevent bending, very light finger pressure is used to retain it in position (Fig. 10–12A and B).

The situation is different in the mandibular arch. Instead of the tori being positioned at the midline, they are seen attached to the lingual side of the mandible and somewhat lateral to the midline. The solution to film positioning lies in the use of a film holder, which allows you to move the film away from the teeth, dropping it down and behind the tori. The increased distance between the film and the teeth is usually not enough to cause significant image distortion (Fig. 10–12C and D).

F. Lingual Frenum Attachment

When the lingual frenum is attached high on the lingual surface of the mandible it interferes with film placement in the anterior mandibular region (Fig. 10–13A and B). Because of the resistance from the frenum, it is not possible to achieve the depth of film placement needed to record the apices of the lower centrals. You have no choice but to place the film on top of the tongue, leaving approximately ⅛

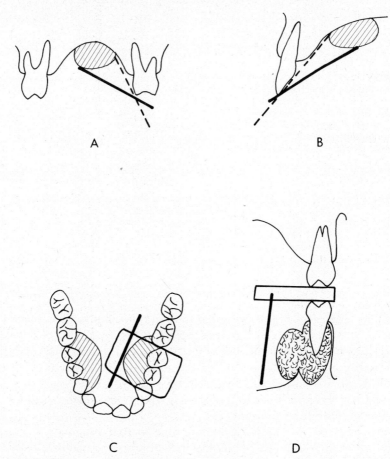

Figure 10–12   *A,* Film placement for a patient with a large maxillary torus (posterior teeth). *Dotted line* = routine placement—will not record root apices. *Solid line* = correct film placement. *B,* Film placement for a patient with a large maxillary torus (anterior teeth). *Dotted line* = routine placement—will not record root apices. *Solid line* = correct film placement. *C,* Occlusal view demonstrating the use of a film holder on a patient with mandibular tori. *D,* Film holder in position for a patient with mandibular tori.

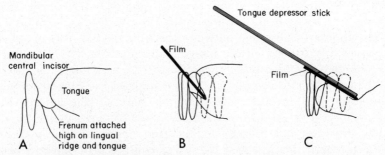

Figure 10–13   *A,* High frenum attachment. *B,* High frenum attachment blocking proper film placement. *C,* Film attached to tongue depressor stick.

inch extending above the incisal edges. Film bending is definitely a problem with finger retention; therefore it is advisable to tape the film to a tongue blade. The patient presses quite hard on top of the tongue blade to decrease the angle formed by the film and the teeth. You may also have to use this procedure for film placement of the cuspids for these patients (Fig. 10–13C).

THE PARALLELING TECHNIQUE

The paralleling technique requires the use of film-holding instruments to establish parallelism between the film and the teeth. These instruments are basically of two types: those which are hand-held by the patient to maintain film position and those which have the patient occlude on the bite-block.

If you can position the film so as to record the apices of the teeth and obtain a reasonable degree of parallelism between the film and teeth, you have basically mastered this technique, as there is no problem in directing the cone perpendicular to the long axis of the teeth.

With these objectives in mind we may now estimate the degree of difficulty anticipated when confronting the following patients:

A. Narrow V-shaped Palate

For this patient there is usually so much difficulty when trying to position the film (even the No. 1 size) that you would save much time and stress by switching over to the short cone and using the bisection of the angle technique. There is a possibility that the mandibular periapicals could be exposed using a film holder, so if you are inclined, give this a try. The difference is that the hard narrow palate will not yield to film pressure, whereas the floor of the mouth may permit the film to be placed deep enough to record the apices. The only other problem in the mandibular arch would be depressing the tongue posteriorly enough to place the film parallel to the anterior teeth. This step is necessary to avoid the narrow constriction of the mandible in the central and cuspid areas.

B. Maxillary Tori

The degree of difficulty encountered in placing the film for the different areas of the maxilla will depend on the size of the torus. With smaller tori, successful film placement is possible. Remember that the film MUST be placed high enough to record the apical region of the teeth, and if bite-block film holders are used the patient MUST occlude on the bite-block when the film is positioned. These last two points are stressed because a large torus will prevent them from being carried out successfully.

Maxillary tori are generally located at the midline or highest part of the palate. When attempting to parallel the film with the teeth, the top edge of the film approximates the midline of the palate. It then becomes obvious that a bony protuberance of any significance would prevent the film from being placed high enough in the palate to record the apices of the teeth. If this problem does arise you have no choice but to replace the long cone with the short cone and bisect the angle. In this case the film will contact the crowns of the teeth and the crest of the torus. For film retention the patient must use very light finger pressure to avoid film bending. The film lies in a more horizontal plane than usual; therefore the vertical angulation will be greater than normal.

C. Mandibular Tori

The mandibular tori are located on the alveolar bone immediately lingual to the teeth and do not present as many problems as maxillary tori. If the tori are located in the bicuspid region, you will not be able to position the film as close to the bicuspids as you would like, but parallelism with the long axis of the teeth can be achieved by dropping the film down and behind the tori. This type of film placement is preferable to laying the film on top of the torus and then bisecting the angle.

When taking radiographs of the centrals and cuspids, it is almost impossible to use a film holder to position the film. If the tori are of any significant size at all, there will be no room between or behind to place the film. Place the film on top of the torus, positioning it as close to normal as possible, and bisect the angle, using either the long or short cone. The mandibular tori do not usually interfere with film placement in the molar area.

When placing the film for a bite-wing exposure, let the film move in toward the tongue. By dropping it down and behind the torus, excessive bending can be prevented. The patient will occlude on the end of the bite-wing tab. Every attempt should be made to place the film anteriorly enough to include the cuspid on the bicuspid bite-wing.

11

THE OCCLUSAL TECHNIQUE

Begin at once to live, and count each day as
a separate life.

Seneca

In addition to the periapical and bite-wing exposures, intraoral occlusal exposures are sometimes necessary. This latter exposure is used to view broader areas of the arch as an aid to diagnosis when there is a cyst, impacted tooth, salivary duct stone, or bone fracture, or for any reason in which the area of interest is larger than that obtained by the periapical technique.

The two most common occlusal views are the anterior view, used to survey the region from cuspid to cuspid, and the cross-section view, which includes the entire arch.

ANTERIOR OCCLUSAL VIEW OF THE MAXILLARY ARCH

A. Adjust the headrest to make the maxillary arch parallel to the floor. The vertical midline of the face should be perpendicular with the floor.

B. Place the occlusal film in the patient's mouth, centering it over the arch. The long axis of the film is placed breadthwise perpendicular to the midline of the arch, and the stippled side of the film is placed against the upper teeth (Fig. 11–1).

C. Instruct the patient to close gently against the film to hold it in position. (If the patient is edentulous, have him use his thumbs to hold the film against the ridge.)

D. The top edge of the cone is placed between the eyebrows at a vertical angulation of +65 degrees. The correct horizontal angulation is obtained by directing the central ray parallel to and through the midline of the arch to the center of the film (Fig. 11–2).

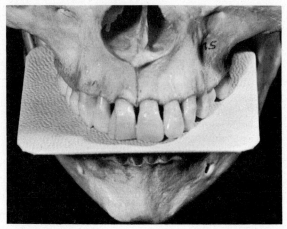

Figure 11–1   Correct position of film for the maxillary occlusal exposure as demonstrated on the skull.

ANTERIOR OCCLUSAL VIEW OF THE MANDIBULAR ARCH

A. Adjust the headrest until the patient's head is tilted back approximately 25 degrees from the vertical.

B. Place the film in the patient's mouth, centering it over the arch. The long axis of the film is placed perpendicular to the midline of the arch, and the stippled side of the film is placed against the lower teeth (Fig. 11–3).

C. Instruct the patient to close gently against the film to hold it in

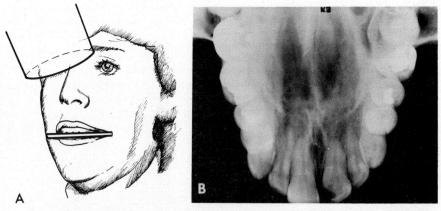

Figure 11–2   *A,* Position of patient, film, and cone tip for the anterior occlusal view of the maxillary arch. *B,* The resultant radiograph.

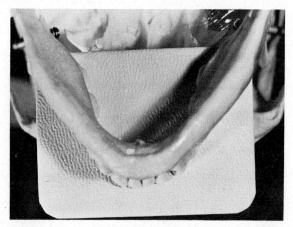

Figure 11–3 Correct position of film for the mandibular occlusal exposure as demonstrated on the skull.

position. (If the patient is edentulous, have him apply pressure with his index fingers to hold the film in position.)

D. Center the cone over the chin at a vertical angulation of −25 degrees. The correct horizontal angulation is obtained by directing the central ray parallel to and through the midline of the arch to the center of the film (Fig. 11–4).

CROSS-SECTION OCCLUSAL VIEW OF THE MAXILLARY ARCH

A. Adjust the headrest to make the maxillary arch parallel to the floor. The vertical midline of the face should be perpendicular to the floor.

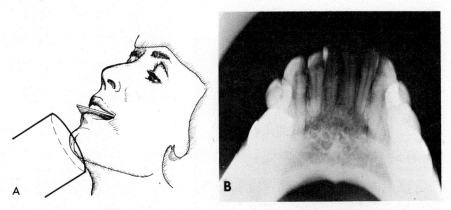

Figure 11–4 *A,* Position of patient, film, and cone tip for the anterior occlusal view of the mandibular arch. *B,* The resultant radiograph.

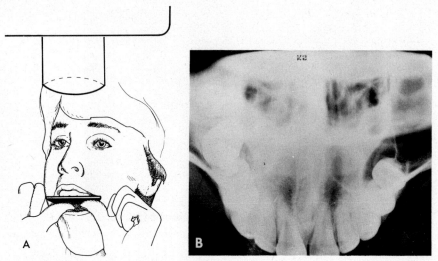

Figure 11–5   *A,* Position of patient, film, and cone tip for the cross-section occlusal view of the maxillary arch. *B,* The resultant radiograph.

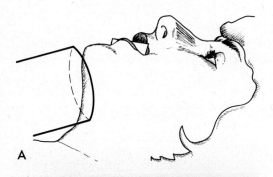

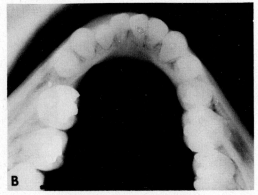

Figure 11–6   *A,* Position of patient, film, and cone tip for the cross-section occlusal view of the mandibular arch. *B,* The resultant radiograph.

B. Place the film in the patient's mouth, centering it over the maxillary arch. The long axis of the film is placed perpendicular to the midline of the arch.

C. Instruct the patient to use his thumbs or to close gently against the film to hold it in place. (If the patient is edentulous, have him hold the film in place with his thumbs.)

D. The edge of the cone is placed at the patient's forehead pointing directly to the center of the film at a 90-degree angle to the film both horizontally and vertically (Fig. 11–5).

CROSS-SECTION OCCLUSAL VIEW OF THE MANDIBULAR ARCH

A. Adjust the headrest so that the patient's head tilts back approximately 75 degrees.

B. Center the occlusal film over the mandibular arch. The long axis of the film should be perpendicular to the midline of the arch. The stippled side of the film is against the lower teeth.

C. Instruct the patient to close on the film to hold it in position. (If the patient is edentulous, have him apply pressure with the index fingers to hold the film in position.)

D. Center the cone approximately 1 inch behind the point of the chin. The central ray should be directed perpendicular to the film both horizontally and vertically (Fig. 11–6).

REMINDERS

1. Always center the film directly over the area of interest so that all needed information can be recorded on the radiograph.
2. Let as little of the film extend beyond the incisal edge of the anterior teeth as possible as this will show up as useless black air space.
3. When going from an upper to a lower occlusal exposure, adjusting the head rest is all that is needed for positioning the patient's head.
4. If a patient is seated in a contoured chair (no adjustable headrest), have him move his head up to a point at which he is looking at the ceiling. This maneuver will facilitate film placement for exposing a lower occlusal film.

12

EXTRAORAL RADIOGRAPHS

Life is too short to be small.

Disraeli

RADIOGRAPHS OF THE DIFFICULT THIRD MOLAR IMPACTIONS

Attempting correct intraoral film placement in many patients can be a trying experience because of the position of the impacted third molar. The third molar placement may cause discomfort or stimulation of the gag reflex. To avoid these problems, the film is placed extraorally in this technique.

With extraoral film placement the x-ray beam must penetrate more tissue (mostly soft tissue), and the resultant radiograph is not as clear as that taken when an intraoral periapical film of the area is exposed. Since it does not have to be used to diagnose decay or other small lesions an extraoral radiograph is quite satisfactory. It should, however, adequately show the third molar impaction and the surrounding structures for observation and surgical purposes. An occlusal film is used to be sure that a broad area surrounding the impaction can be observed.

IMPACTED LOWER THIRD MOLAR EXPOSURE

A. Adjust the headrest so that the maxillary arch is parallel to the floor.

B. Place the film horizontally (long axis parallel to the floor), with the lower edge parallel to and even with the lower border of the mandible, centering it over the impacted tooth. (The third molar can be located by observing an intraoral exposure of the mandibular second molar area. Even though only a portion of the crown may be seen, this is sufficient to determine its position.)

C. Instruct the patient to hold the film in this position (Fig. 12–1).

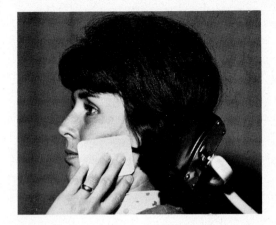

Figure 12–1 Film placement for impacted lower third molar.

D. Have the patient "push her chin away from her neck" while maintaining the back of her head firmly in the headrest to prevent movement during the exposure. Extending the chin separates the mandible from the vertebrae and eliminates the possibility of superimposing the vertebrae over the impaction. To help the patient assume this position, stand in front of her, placing your left hand on top of her head and the fingers of your right hand under her chin, exerting a pulling action toward you with your right hand. After extension of the chin, tilt her head approximately 10 degrees toward the side on which the film is held.

E. Locate the angle of the mandible opposite the side being exposed by palpating the area with your fingers. Place the cone tip just inferior and posterior to this angle, keeping in mind that the central rays must pass slightly under this angle to prevent superimposition of one side of the mandible over the other. Point the central ray through the tissues of the neck to the impaction. It is impossible to direct it perpendicular to the film in a vertical direction owing to the tilting of the head. Therefore some minor degree of elongation of the structures on the film is unavoidable. For horizontal angulation the ray is directed perpendicular to the flat surface of the film (Fig. 12–2).

F. Instruct the patient to maintain her teeth in occlusion during the exposure taken at 90 k.v.p. − 15 ma. − 1 sec. (Fig. 12–3).

An exposure of the upper third molar can be taken by making a few minor changes in this technique. The following procedure will also successfully expose both upper and lower impactions on one film. In positioning the patient follow the same procedure as for the lower impaction, making sure that the head is extended from the neck. To complete the setup two changes are necessary. (1) The occlusal film is placed vertically so that the upper half of the film is centered directly over the impacted maxillary third molar. Again, the inferior edge of the film is parallel to and even with the inferior border of the mandible

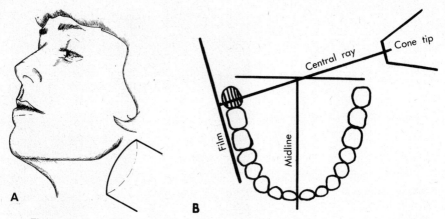

Figure 12–2 *A*, Placement of cone tip for impacted lower third molar. *B*, Diagram indicating direction of central ray.

(Fig. 12–4). (2) To reduce vertical distortion (elongation) of the upper third molar impaction, the center of the cone is placed approximately 1 inch above the angle of the mandible and just posterior to the posterior border of the mandible. The central rays are directed to the center of an imaginary line connecting the upper and lower third molars (Fig. 12–5).

LATERAL JAW EXPOSURE

A similar technique to the one just described is known as the lateral jaw projection. It is used to show broader areas of the mandible,

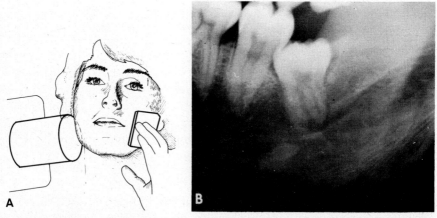

Figure 12–3 *A*, Placement of patient, film, and cone tip for impacted lower third molar. *B*, Resultant radiograph.

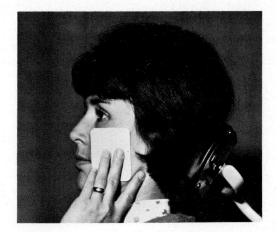

Figure 12–4 Film placement for impacted upper third molar.

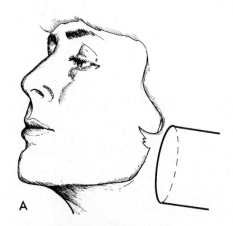

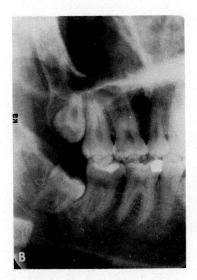

Figure 12–5 *A,* Placement of cone tip for impacted upper third molar. *B,* Resultant radiograph.

and it includes the posterior portion of the maxilla as well. Conditions which call for this exposure are the presence of large cystic lesions, one or more impacted teeth, the suspicion of a fracture, or patients who cannot open their mouths for placement of intraoral films.

A 5 × 7 inch film is used. Owing to the small amount of bone to be penetrated, a nonscreen film in a film holder is sufficient; however, a screen film in a cassette may also be used.

Positioning of the patient is just the same as that for taking the radiograph of an impacted lower third molar. The film is placed horizontally over the mandible and centered over the first molar (Fig. 12–6). The lower edge of the film is parallel to and even with the inferior border of the mandible. The exception to the previously described technique is in the placement of the tube head. Although the horizontal and vertical angulations are adjusted in the same manner as that for the impacted lower third molar, the cone is placed approximately 5 inches from the patient. This increase in the tube-film distance provides a greater area of radiation at the film to adequately expose the larger area of the 5 × 7 film (Fig. 12–7). With nonscreen film, the exposure is taken at 65 k.v.p. − 10 ma. − 1.5 sec.

PANORAMIC X-RAY UNITS

The panoramic unit takes extraoral radiographs of both maxillary and mandibular arches with one exposure. The Panorex (S.S. White

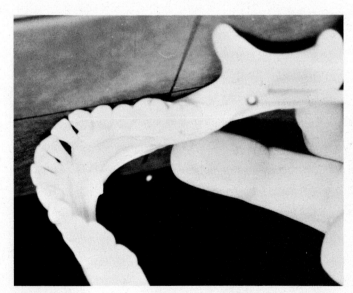

Figure 12–6 Relative position of mandible to the film holder as seen from the top view.

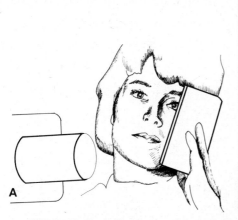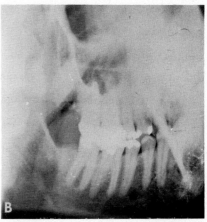

Figure 12–7 A, Placement of patient, film, and cone tip for lateral jaw exposure. B, Resultant radiograph.

Dental Mfg. Co., X.R.M. Division) is shown in Figure 12–8. A radiograph of this type (Fig. 12–9) is most useful in orthodontics because it exhibits the spacing and the crowding of the teeth and the growth pattern of both jaws; in surgery because it exhibits impacted third molars, fractures of the mandible, and the complete outline of any pathological lesions when present; and in periodontics because it exhibits the condition of the bone supporting the teeth. There is some loss of detail in the radiograph because the Panorex film is exposed outside the patient's mouth (extraorally). The detail is adequate, however, for the purposes given.

When taking a panoramic exposure, the x-ray tube head and the cassette holder rotate around the patient's head during the operational cycle. The cassette, which occupies one half of the cassette holder, moves to the other half of the holder in synchronization with the movement of the tube head as it circles the patient's head. Midway during the cycle the chair shifts approximately 2 inches to one side to change the axis of rotation (Fig. 12–12). The chair movement reduces the amount of film image distortion. Though the exposure takes approximately 20 seconds to completion, the patient receives only 0.8 r of radiation. The x-rays come through the tube head from a narrow line opening, giving the x-ray beam a narrow band shape instead of the conventional cone-shaped beam. Consequently, much less tissue is irradiated as the beam passes through the patient to the film. Film is manufactured specifically for these units.

Another type of panoramic unit is the Panelipse (General Electric Co., Medical Systems Division). (See Fig. 12–10.) This unit operates in a manner similar to that described above. It uses a flexible cassette

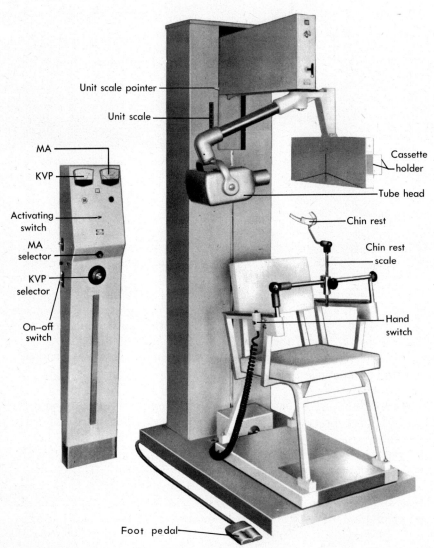

Unit scale pointer

Unit scale

MA

KVP

Activating switch

MA selector

KVP selector

On–off switch

Cassette holder

Tube head

Chin rest

Chin rest scale

Hand switch

Foot pedal

Figure 12–8 Panoramic x-ray unit. (Courtesy of the S. S. White Dental Mfg. Co., X.R.M. Division.)

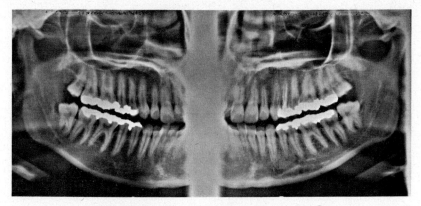

Figure 12–9 Panoramic radiograph of an adult.

loaded on a film drum. The film drum rotates in coordination with the movement of the tube head as it moves around the patient's head (Fig. 12–11). With this unit there is no shifting of the chair at the midpoint of the exposure. The resultant film therefore shows a continuous image.

Procedure

A. The film is placed in a cassette secured with spring clamps, then placed in the cassette holder (Fig. 12–13).

B. Before the patient is seated, a caliper is used to determine the approximate width of the patient's head. Refer to the chart provided which will determine the KVP setting and a corresponding MA setting for each respective patient.

C. The patient is seated and his chin placed in the chin rest so that the head is positioned symmetrically (Fig. 12–14). The maxillary arch should tilt down approximately 10 degrees from the horizontal plane. If the patient's head is not exactly centered in the chin rest, the molars on the resultant film will be unequal in size. When the patient is positioned in accordance with these instructions, the spinal column will be located directly behind his central incisors.

D. If you wish to prevent vertical overlapping of the teeth, a cotton roll may be placed between the patient's incisors.

E. The cassette and tube head must be in direct alignment with the patient's arches. To accomplish this, raise or lower the tube head by means of the foot pedal and hand switch until the number on the chin rest scale matches that on the unit scale (Fig. 12–15).

F. Always explain to the patient what to expect during the ex-

Text continued on page 149.

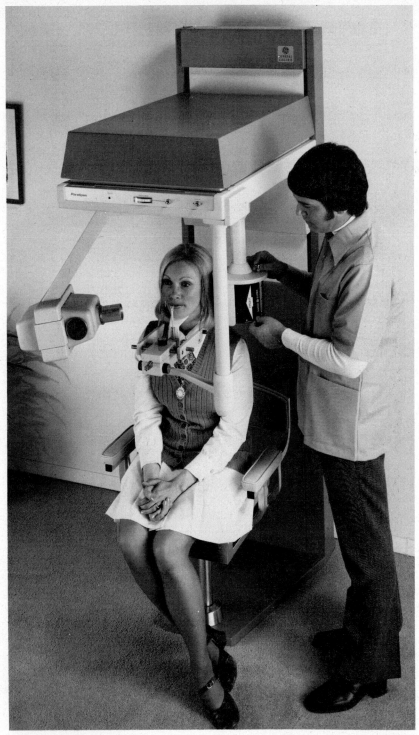

Figure 12–10 Panelipse panoramic x-ray unit. (Courtesy of the General Electric Co., Medical Systems Division.)

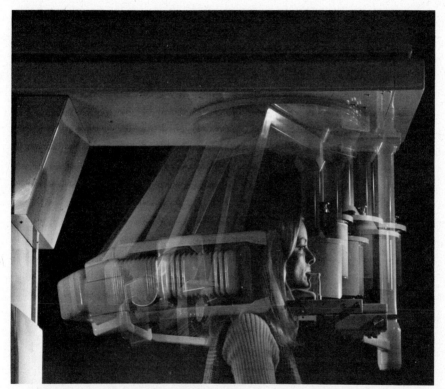

Figure 12–11   Rotation of the Panelipse x-ray unit. (Courtesy of the General Electric Co., Medical Systems Division.)

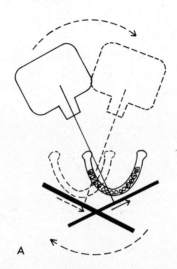

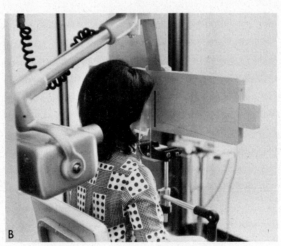

Figure 12–12 *A,* Schematic drawing of the tube head and cassette holder at the midpoint of the exposure. Note the shift in the mandible representing the shift of the chair. The small arrows indicate the movement of the film past the slit opening in the cassette holder. The large arrows indicate the movement of the tube head and the cassette holder around the patient's head. *B,* Position of cassette holder and tube head at midpoint when the chair shifts.

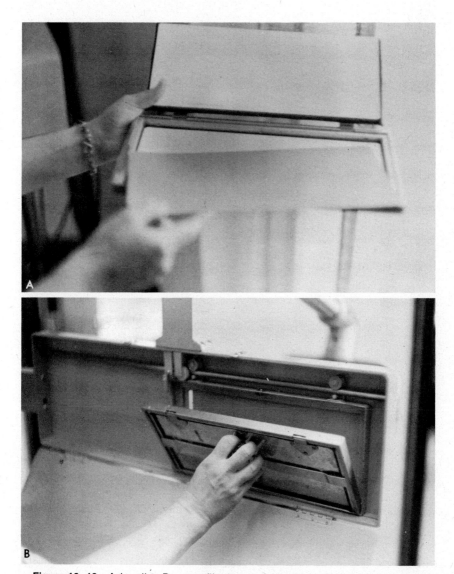

Figure 12–13 *A*, Loading Panorex film into cassette (to be done in dark room only). *B*, Placing cassette into cassette holder of unit.

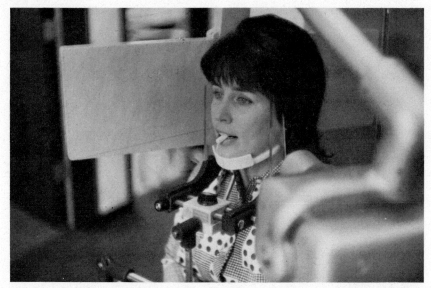

Figure 12–14 Positioning of patient's head in chin rest.

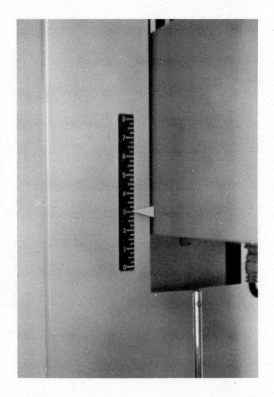

Figure 12–15 The unit scale, which must correspond to the number on the chin rest scale.

posure, specifically: (1) The cassette and tube head will rotate around his head. (2) At the midway point, the chair will move approximately 2 inches. (3) The exposure time is 20 seconds, throughout which the patient must remain completely still.

REMINDERS

When exposing extraoral radiographs of third molars:

1. Do not position the film too far posteriorly when placing it vertically to record both upper and lower third molars.
2. No part of the film should extend below the inferior border of the mandible.
3. The film should be held flat against the face.
4. The central ray is directed from behind the mandible forward to the film (Fig. 12–2*B*).

13

THE CHILD PATIENT

Observe all men; thyself most.

Ben Franklin

The technical procedure for taking radiographs of children is essentially the same as that for adults. However, you will obviously be working in an area of greater confinement, and occasionally the behavior problem can make the x-ray procedure more difficult.

From birth through 6 years of age the formation and development of the child's teeth and facial bones are taking place at a rapid rate (Fig. 13-1). Children in this age bracket are usually referred to as preschool children, and it is during this period that the child should have his first dental check-up.

Radiographs of the child are a necessity if a complete and thorough diagnosis is to be made. The roots of erupted primary teeth as well as the developing permanent teeth located within the confines of the alveolar bone are seen on these radiographs. So much development is taking place underneath the surface of the gingivae that this is the only means of accurately examining this area. In addition, many carious lesions, which are quite prevalent in this age bracket, are overlooked without a radiograph. These lesions can be detected with a mouth mirror and an explorer only after they have inflicted extensive damage to the structure of the tooth. A radiograph can demonstrate interproximal lesions in the beginning stages so that they can be removed before the tooth is placed in jeopardy.

Without a radiograph it is possible that up to 50 per cent of the total number of lesions may be overlooked. This is reason enough to make an x-ray examination an absolute necessity during these early years.

Disturbances in the normal developmental processes generally can be diagnosed only through adequate radiographs. As a child becomes older, a permanent tooth may not erupt within normal time limits. Is it missing? Is it being blocked in its normal eruptive path? Is it malposed or impacted? These questions can only be answered by a radiograph. Also, periapical infection and other disease processes are clarified and diagnosed by viewing a radiograph of the area in question.

Quite frequently children injure their teeth in a fall or by a blow to the mouth. The extent of damage to the teeth, supporting bone, and periapical tissues as a result of the trauma needs the clarification of a radiograph.

Unless an emergency dictates, the child is usually seen for his first routine dental check when he is about 3 years old. His first visit to the dental office should be a pleasant one. Greet him personally and escort him into the operatory. Parents should remain in the waiting room, because the child will adapt to this new experience more readily when a sympathetic mother or father is not present.

After he is seated in the dental chair, establish rapport with him by discussing such personal subjects as his age, interests, and family, and by complimenting him on his appearance or clothes. Before proceeding with the radiographic examination, explain to him in terms he can understand what you are about to do. Show him the film, let him handle it, and describe the x-ray unit as a camera that will take pictures of his teeth. Showing him the "pictures" of other children's teeth may also be helpful.

When you encounter a refractory child, be firm and let him know you are in command of the situation. If he still offers resistance, or if he has refused to enter the operatory alone, it may be helpful for the parent to be present during this first visit. In any case do not physically force him to cooperate, as this might instill in him a fear of dentistry that he may never overcome.

The most satisfactory radiographs are the intraoral bite-wings of the posterior teeth and periapical exposures of all areas of both arches (Fig. 13-2). An attempt should be made to take this complete series of radiographs. However, intraoral film placement in some very young patients is often not worth the time-consuming persuasive effort it requires. Frequent problems, for both periapical and bite-wing exposures, are resistance to film placement by the tongue and stimulation of the gag reflex. Rather than reaching a diagnosis from clinical examination alone, a correctly exposed lateral jaw film can supply much needed information; the extraoral film placement that it requires is not objectionable to most children. It is possible to detect interproximal caries in this exposure and to observe tooth relationships and arch development. Also observable are both the primary posterior teeth and the developing permanent posterior teeth.

When the lateral jaw exposures are taken in place of the periapical series, occlusal films of both arches are necessary as well. Most children offer no resistance to the intraoral placement of the occlusal film. Following the lateral jaw and occlusal exposures, the child should be

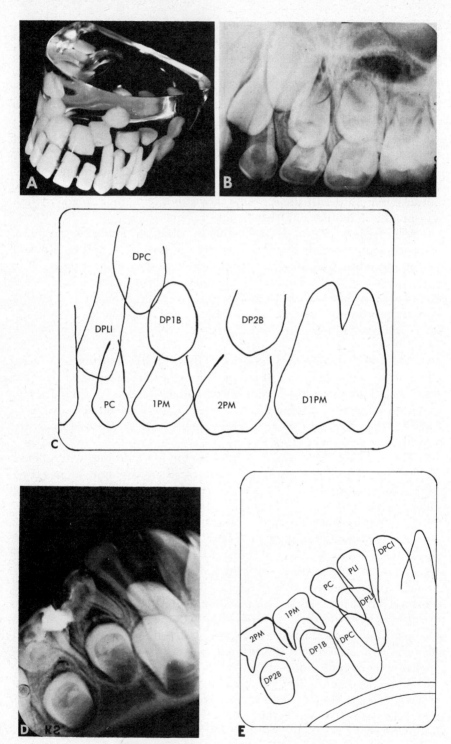

Figure 13–1 See legend on opposite page.

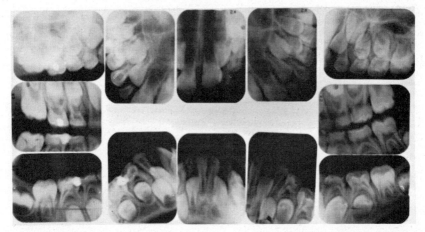

Figure 13-2 A mounted series of periapical and bite-wing radiographs demonstrating each area of tooth development.

"warming up" to the radiographic procedure. At this time the bite-wing exposures can usually be taken, since the child has gained confidence from the previous exposures. Success in taking these six films provides a most satisfactory replacement for the complete intraoral series.

By the time a child is 6 years old, his reasoning capacity and maturity have usually increased to the point that periapical and bite-wing exposures with No. 2 film can be tolerated. This patient will usually exhibit a mixed dentition with the loss of the primary anterior teeth that have been followed by the eruption of the permanent central and lateral incisors and permanent first molars. By the age of 10 to 12, the permanent cuspids and bicuspids will be erupting into their respective positions. At any time during this period a lateral jaw exposure will give an overall view of the developmental and eruptive stages of the permanent posterior teeth. When the child has reached the age of 12, the second permanent molars should be making their appearance. At

---

Figure 13-1 *A,* A plastic model showing the relationship of the developing permanent teeth to the erupted primary teeth. On a radiograph this relationship will be the same. *B* and *C,* A radiograph and diagrammatic sketch of the maxillary posterior region showing the relationship of the developing permanent teeth to the erupted primary teeth. *D* and *E,* A radiograph and diagrammatic sketch of the mandibular cuspid region showing the relationship of the developing permanent teeth to the erupted primary teeth.

Key to Parts *C* and *E:*

PLI = primary lateral incisor
PC = primary cuspid
1PM = first primary molar
2PM = second primary molar
DPCI = developing permanent central
    incisor
DPLI = developing permanent lateral
    incisor

DPC = developing permanent cuspid
DP1B = developing permanent first
    bicuspid
DP2B = developing permanent second
    bicuspid
D1PM = developing first permanent
    molar

this age the child should be considered an adult as far as the radiographic procedure is concerned.

The following is the list of exposures generally used according to the age of the child.

Up to age 6:   *Preferred*
Ten periapical exposures, including (in each arch) a central-lateral incisor exposure, right and left cuspid exposures, and right and left molar exposures.
A posterior bite-wing of each side.
Alternate
A lateral jaw exposure of each side.
An occlusal film of each arch.
A posterior bite-wing of each side.

Ages 6 to 12:   Ten periapical exposures, including (in each arch) a central-lateral incisor exposure, right and left cuspid exposures, and right and left molar exposures.
A posterior bite-wing of each side.

PERIAPICAL AND BITE-WING EXPOSURES

The procedures for taking the periapical and bite-wing exposures in the child are the same as for the adult patient, with just minor changes to compensate for a child's smaller arch.

There are two sizes of film used for children: the routine adult periapical film (No. 2), and the smaller children's film (No. 1). Whenever possible use the larger film, for it provides more area coverage for diagnostic information.

The placement of the film is the same as that for the adult, but a child with deciduous teeth and 6-year molars will not need as many exposures as an older child with erupted 12-year molars. Because the smaller size film is more adaptable to the oral tissues, for periapical exposures it will lie more in line with the long axis of the teeth. The larger film tends to lie in a more horizontal position, which increases the angle formed by the teeth and the film. Therefore, when using the bisection of the angle technique, the vertical angulation will be increased for most exposures, with the exception of the bite-wing exposures, in comparison to the angulation necessary in the same exposures of an adult.

Following are brief descriptions of the procedures, with the changes necessary for taking radiographs of children. The film should be maintained in position with the thumb for maxillary exposures and

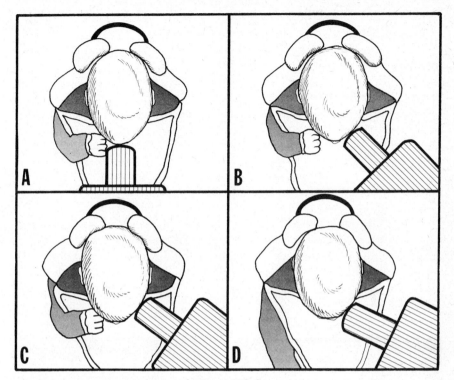

Figure 13–3

with the index finger for mandibular exposures. For purposes of demonstration, the film used in the photographs that show film placement on the study model of a child is the No. 0 size. Figure 13–3A to D demonstrates the horizontal angulations for each exposure.

Maxillary Arch

Central-Lateral Incisor Exposure (**Fig. 13–4A**).   The film is placed vertically and centered over the two central incisors with approximately ⅛ inch extending below and parallel to the incisal edge. The resultant exposure should show the maxillary central and lateral incisors and the adjacent area.

Cuspid Exposure (**Fig. 13–4B**).   The film is centered vertically over the cuspid in the same manner as for the adult. If it cannot be placed so that the inferior edge is parallel to the incisal edge of the teeth, an oblique placement will suffice. In either case, approximately

⅛ inch of the film should extend below the edge of the teeth. This exposure will show the cuspid and adjacent area.

Posterior Exposure **(Fig. 13–4C).** Until the permanent second molars erupt, only one exposure of the posterior area is necessary. This should adequately show the primary molars and the permanent first molars. The film is centered over the posterior teeth with approximately ⅛ inch below the occlusal edge. This exposure, if positioned correctly, will show part of the cuspid and both the primary molars and permanent first molars.

Posterior Bite-Wing Exposure (Fig. 13–4D)

One bite-wing on each side is all that is necessary to adequately expose the crowns of the posterior teeth. The film is softened at the anterior corners and then centered over the lower posterior teeth. Instruct the child to close slowly while rolling your finger to the side of

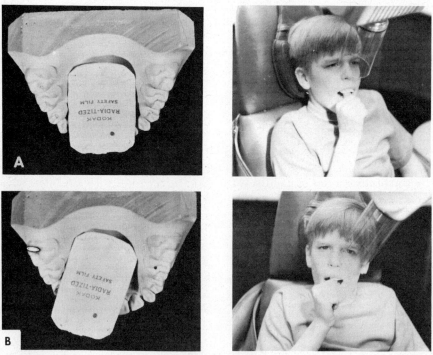

Figure 13–4 Correct film placement demonstrated on a plaster model and correct position of the patient, film, and cone for the following exposures:
A, Maxillary central-lateral exposure.
B, Maxillary cuspid exposure.

Illustration continues on opposite page.

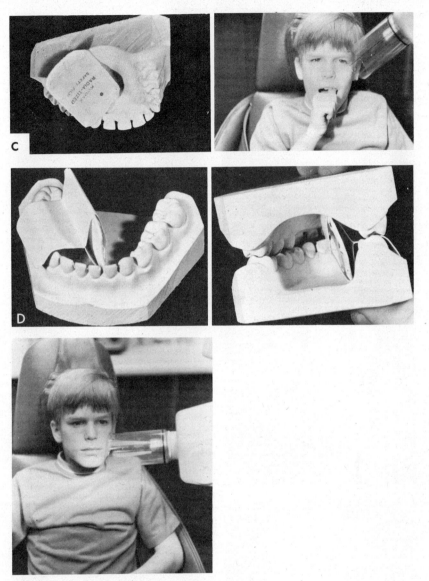

Figure 13–4 *Continued.*
C, Maxillary posterior exposure.
D, Posterior bite-wing exposure. Posterior view of plaster model shows the film being held in position as the patient closes on the bite-wing tab. (X-ray unit courtesy of the General Electric Co., X-ray Department.)

the teeth. When the teeth are closed on the tab the film will be maintained in position.

Owing to the curvature of the palate, the upper half of the film will bend slightly to conform to this curvature. To compensate for this, the vertical angulation should be set at +10 degrees.

Mandibular Arch

Central-Lateral Incisor Exposure (**Fig. 13–5A**). Place the film vertically underneath the tongue so that it is centered over the two central incisors. Every attempt should be made to place the film deep enough so that approximately ⅛ inch is above and parallel to the incisal edge.

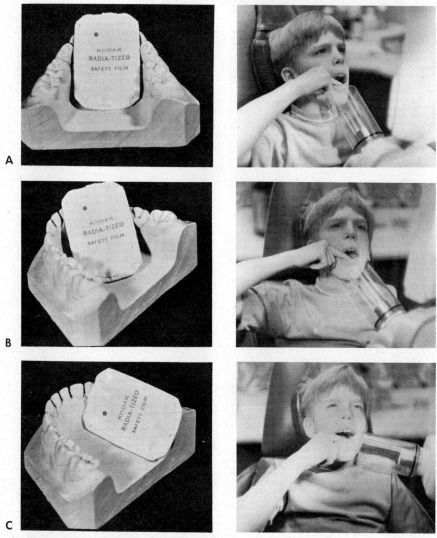

Figure 13–5 Correct film placement demonstrated on a plaster model and correct position of the patient, film, and cone for the following exposures:

A, Mandibular central-lateral exposure.

B, Mandibular cuspid exposure.

C, Mandibular posterior exposure.

(X-ray unit courtesy of the General Electric Co., X-ray Department.)

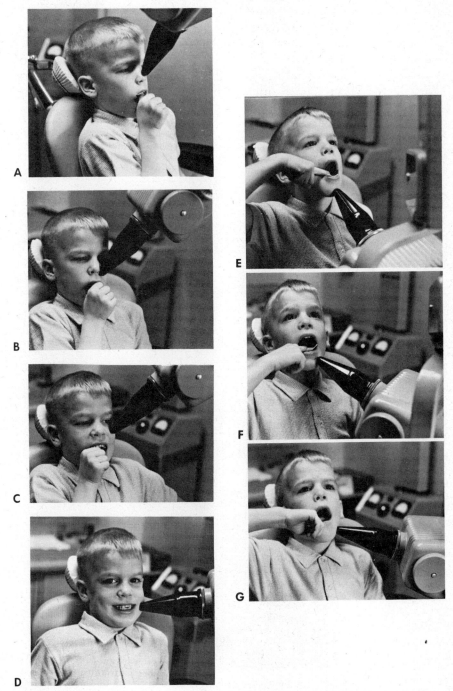

Figure 13-6   Film, patient, and cone tip positioning when using the pointed plastic cone. *A,* Maxillary centrals and laterals. *B,* Maxillary cuspids. *C,* Maxillary posteriors. *D,* Posterior bite-wing. *E,* Mandibular centrals and laterals. *F,* Mandibular cuspids. *G,* Mandibular posteriors.

As with the maxillary exposure, you will see the central and lateral incisors and adjacent area on the resultant radiograph.

Cuspid Exposure (**Fig. 13–5B**). Place the film vertically underneath the tongue so that it is centered over the cuspid. Approximately ⅛ inch of the film should extend above and be parallel to the incisal edge of the teeth. The resultant exposure will show the cuspid and surrounding area.

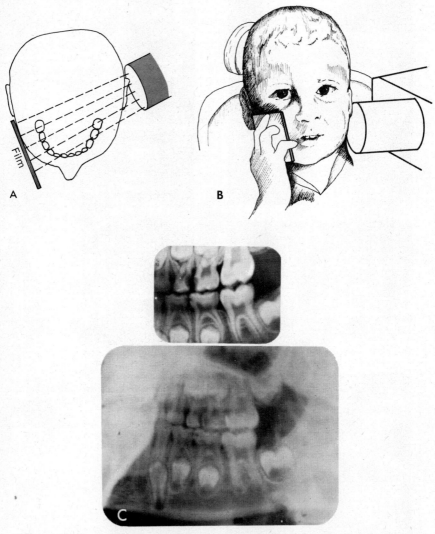

Figure 13–7 *A* and *B*, Lateral jaw exposure. *A*, Diagrammatic sketch of the top view of the patient, illustrating horizontal angulation. *B*, Correct position of the patient, film, and cone tip (vertical angulation). *C*, Comparison of a lateral jaw exposure with an intraoral bite-wing exposure (top) of the same teeth. Interproximal caries can be detected on both exposures between the mandibular first and second primary molars.

Posterior Exposure (**Fig. 13–5C**).   Until the second permanent molar has erupted, one exposure is all that is necessary to adequately show the primary molars and permanent first molars. The film is centered over the posterior teeth with ⅛ inch above and parallel to the occlusal edge of the teeth.

LATERAL JAW EXPOSURES (Figs. 13–7 and 13–8)

Adjust the child's head by making the upper arch parallel to the floor, and then tilt the head slightly toward the side to be exposed. Have the child clench his teeth lightly as you center the film over the posterior teeth of both arches. The inferior edge of the film should be even with the inferior border of the mandible. Then instruct the child to place his fingers against the film to hold it in this position. The tube head is then adjusted so that the central ray passes from just behind the angle of the mandible at a −5 to −10 degree vertical angulation to the center of the film. The cone tip should just touch the surface of the skin.

OCCLUSAL EXPOSURES

Anterior Exposure of the Maxillary Arch (**Fig. 13–9**).   Adjust the headrest so that the child's head is upright and the maxillary arch is parallel to the floor. Place an adult-size periapical film in the mouth,

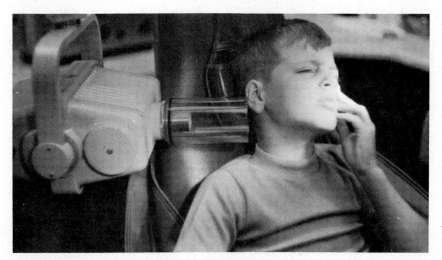

Figure 13–8   Position of film, patient, and cone tip when using the open end short cone to take a radiograph of the lateral jaw exposure.

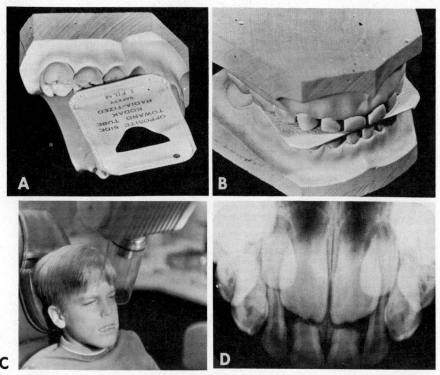

Figure 13–9 Anterior maxillary occlusal exposure. *A* and *B*, Correct film placement demonstrated on plaster models. *C*, Correct position of the patient, film, and cone for this exposure. *D*, Resultant radiograph.

pebbled side up, with the anterior edge of the film even with the incisal edges of the central incisors. Instruct the child to close on the film. The cone is placed between the eyebrows, with the central ray directed to the center of the film at a +65 degree vertical angulation. To show a larger area of the maxilla, an occlusal film, rather than the periapical film, may be used. It is placed in a lengthwise position and is centered over the arch.

Anterior Exposure of the Mandibular Arch (**Fig. 13–10**). Adjust the headrest until the child's head tilts back at an angle of 25 degrees from the vertical. The film is placed in the mouth with the pebbled side down and the anterior edge even with the incisal edges of the lower central incisors. Instruct the child to close on the film. The center of the cone is placed at the point of the chin at a vertical angulation of −25 degrees. As in the maxillary exposure, an occlusal film may be used to show a larger area. (Use same exposure time as for periapical exposures.)

Cross-Section Exposure of the Maxillary Arch (**Fig. 13–11A and**

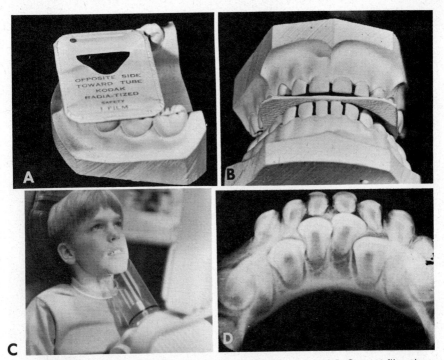

Figure 13–10 Anterior mandibular occlusal exposure. *A* and *B*, Correct film place-ment demonstrated on plaster models. *C*, Correct position of the patient, film, and cone for this exposure. *D*, Resultant radiograph.

B).   The headrest is adjusted so that the maxillary arch is parallel to the floor. An intraoral cassette containing the occlusal film is placed, tube side up, as far posterior in the mouth as possible. It is held in this position with thumb pressure. The edge of the cone is positioned at the child's forehead with the central ray directed at an angle of 90 degrees to the center of the cassette (90 k.v.p. − 15 ma. − 1 sec.).

Cross-Section Exposure of the Mandibular Arch (**Fig. 13–11C and D**).   The headrest is adjusted so that the child's head tilts back at an angle of 45 degrees. Place an occlusal film, pebbled side down, as far posterior in the mouth as possible. Instruct the child to close on the film to maintain it in this position. The center of the cone is placed at a point 1 inch posterior from the tip of the chin, with the tube head angled at −45 degrees. The central ray will then be directed to the center of the film at an angle of 90 degrees to the film (65 k.v.p. − 10 ma. − 0.5 sec.).

Bite-Wing Exposures (**Up to Age 6**).   These are taken in the same manner as for adults (Fig. 13–12).

Panorex Exposures.   A panoramic view of both arches of the child

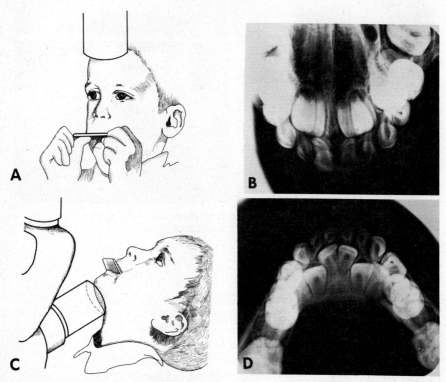

Figure 13–11   Cross-section occlusal exposures. *A,* Correct position of the patient, film, and cone for the maxillary cross-section occlusal exposure. *B,* Resultant radiograph. *C,* Correct position of the patient, film, and cone for the mandibular cross-section occlusal exposure. *D,* Resultant radiograph.

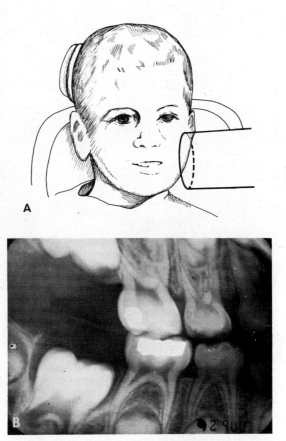

Figure 13–12   Bite-wing exposure of a young child. *A,* Correct position of the patient, film, and cone for this exposure. *B,* Resultant radiograph.

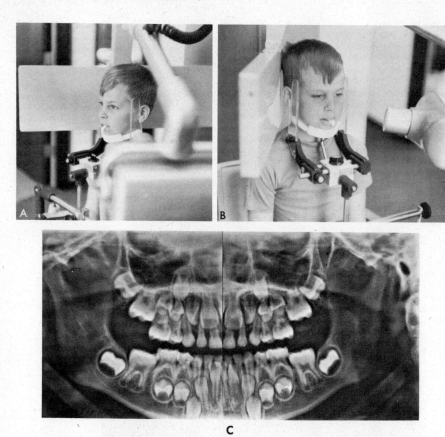

Figure 13–13 *A* and *B*, Positioning of Panorex unit for x-raying the child patient. Note cotton roll placed to prevent vertical overlap of teeth on resultant radiograph. *C*, Panoramic radiograph of a young child.

is an excellent supplement to the previous exposures, especially for viewing overall jaw development and developing permanent teeth (Fig. 13–13).

REMINDERS

1. Tell children how much they are helping you when they hold the film in position. Involve them as much as possible and use PRAISE.
2. Some children need to be handled firmly. If necessary, do so. Once they know YOU are the boss of the situation, a smoother x-ray procedure usually results.
3. Considerable softening of bite-wing films will make occlusion on the tab much easier.
4. Once film is positioned, move fast.

14

THE EDENTULOUS PATIENT

*Not in doing what you like but in liking what
you do is the secret of happiness.*

J. M. Barrie

The ridges of most edentulous patients present a normal appearance which may cause a laxity in procuring radiographs of the arches to accompany the clinical examination. But before a denture is fabricated, the dentist must be satisfied in his own mind that these edentulous areas are normal and healthy. That is why good radiographs of these patients are a necessity.

When confronted with a fully or partially edentulous patient you must remember that the patient once had the normal complement of teeth in both arches. Why are these teeth now missing? Some of these patients were no doubt involved in unfortunate accidents in which many teeth were lost, but in the majority of cases the teeth were lost through the patient's negligence. The process of decay accounts for much of the loss, but in many instances perfectly good teeth have to be extracted because advanced periodontal disease destroyed the supporting bone. The infectious processes, resulting from excessively decayed teeth or advanced periodontal disease, developed in what are now the edentulous ridges. Though the teeth are now absent, the question must be resolved as to whether the infectious process is still present. The radiographs will answer this, as well as detecting previously overlooked root tips, unerupted teeth, abnormal changes of bone, cysts, and so on.

In general the basic rules of the bisection of the angle technique are followed when exposing roentgenographs of the edentulous patient. However, there is necessarily a change in the angulation of the film placement and of the tube head. The area of interest is the ridge proper of the arches instead of the teeth and supporting structures (Fig. 14–1).

Periapical films are used; although the teeth are absent, the full series is the same as for the dentulous patient. The exposures for both

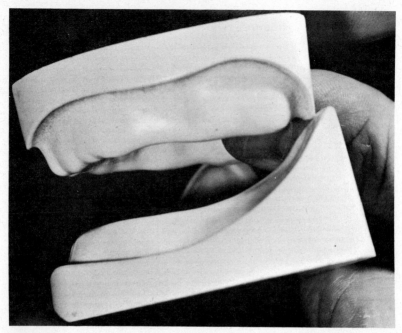

Figure 14-1 Plaster model of edentulous ridges showing the approximate relationship of the maxillary and mandibular arches.

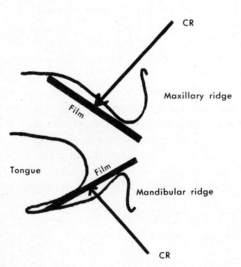

Figure 14-2 Diagram showing film in position in the edentulous patient and approximate vertical angulation.

the mandibular and maxillary arches are the central-lateral incisor area, the cuspid area, the bicuspid-molar area, and the third molar area. The bite-wing exposures for detection of caries are, of course, eliminated.

The procedure to be followed is the same as that set forth in Chapters 5 and 6. After the patient's head is correctly positioned, the film is inserted in the mouth. When placing the films in a mouth with prominent ridges, no more than 1/4 inch of the film should extend above the mandibular arch or below the maxillary arch. The film is placed vertically for anterior exposures and horizontally for posterior ones. The patient is instructed to hold the film in position in the same manner as the dentulous patient, i.e., with the thumb for all maxillary exposures and with the index finger for all mandibular exposures.

The vertical angulation is adjusted according to the bisection of the angle method. In place of the longitudinal axis of the tooth, a vertical

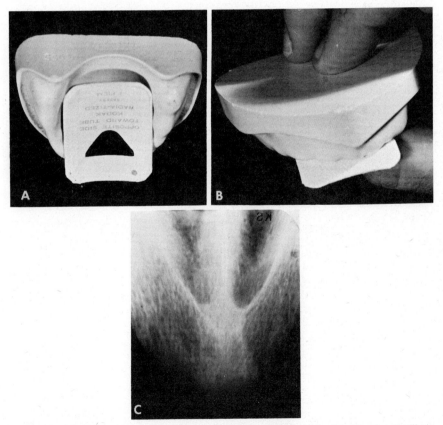

Figure 14–3   Maxillary central incisor area. *A* and *B,* The film is placed vertically in the mouth so that the midline of the film is directly over the midline of the arch. Approximately 1/4 inch of the film extends below the crest of the ridge. *C,* Resultant radiograph.

line through the ridge forms one side of the angle and the film forms the other. After the correct vertical angulation is established, direct the central rays to the center of the film (Fig. 14-2).

Determination of the horizontal angulation is not so critical, because there is no need to avoid overlapping of the teeth on the resultant radiograph. In this case the angulation is adjusted by directing the central ray perpendicular to the horizontal plane of the film.

When you encounter a patient with extremely small ridges, or with no ridges at all, the angle of film placement changes considerably. In all but the mandibular molar area, the film will be almost parallel to the floor. The vertical angulation is much increased to compensate for this, so that it is in almost the same position as when an occlusal film is exposed.

The same series of film placements is followed. Every attempt

Text continued on page 178.

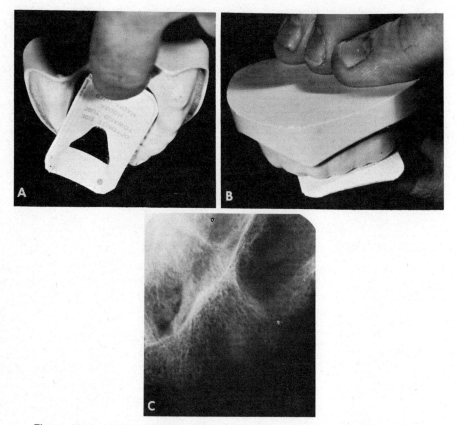

Figure 14-4 Maxillary cuspid area. *A* and *B,* The film is placed vertically in the mouth over the cuspid area. Approximately ¼ inch of the film extends below the crest of the ridge. *C,* Resultant radiograph.

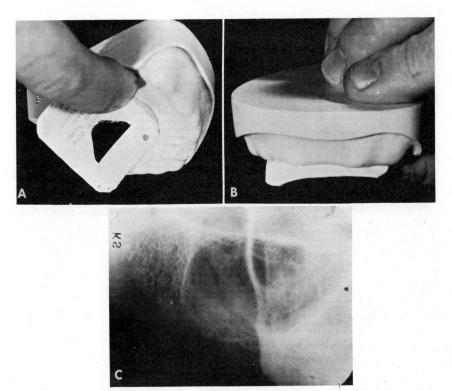

Figure 14–5   Maxillary bicuspid-molar area. *A* and *B*, The film is placed horizontally in the mouth over the bicuspid-first molar area. Approximately ¼ inch of the film extends below the crest of the ridge. *C*, Resultant radiograph.

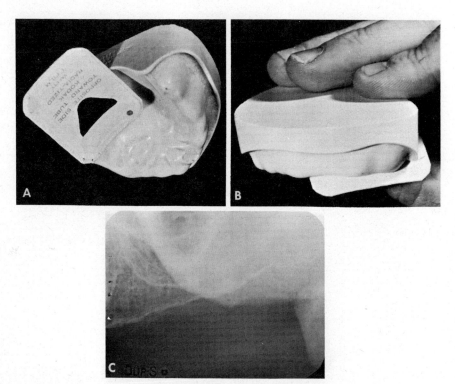

Figure 14-6 Maxillary tuberosity area. *A* and *B*, The film is placed horizontally in the mouth and centered over the maxillary tuberosity. Approximately ¼ inch of the film extends below the crest of the ridge. *C*, Resultant radiograph.

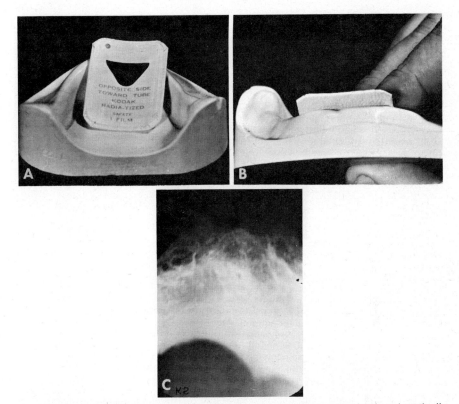

Figure 14–7   Mandibular central incisor area. *A* and *B,* The film is placed vertically in the mouth so that the midline of the film is directly over the midline of the arch. Approximately ¼ inch of the film extends above the crest of the ridge. *C,* Resultant radiograph.

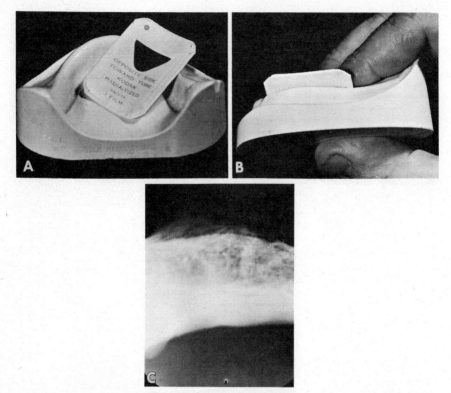

Figure 14–8 Mandibular cuspid area. *A* and *B*, The film is placed vertically in the mouth over the cuspid area. Approximately ¼ inch of the film extends above the crest of the ridge. *C*, Resultant radiograph.

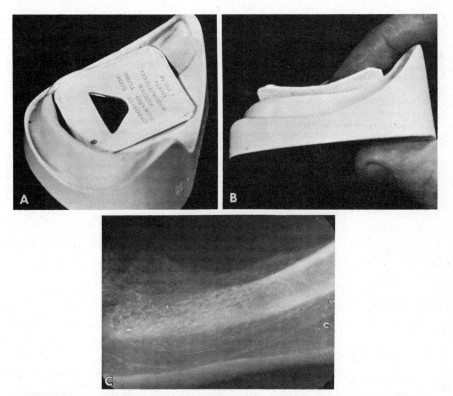

Figure 14–9 Mandibular bicuspid-molar area. *A* and *B,* The film is placed horizontally in the mouth and centered over the bicuspid–first molar area. Approximately ¼ inch of the film extends above the crest of the ridge. *C,* Resultant radiograph.

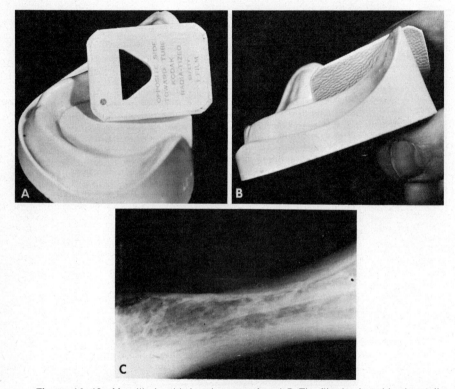

Figure 14–10 Mandibular third molar area. *A* and *B*, The film is placed horizontally in the mouth and centered over the third molar area. Approximately ¼ inch of the film extends above the crest of the ridge. *C*, Resultant radiograph.

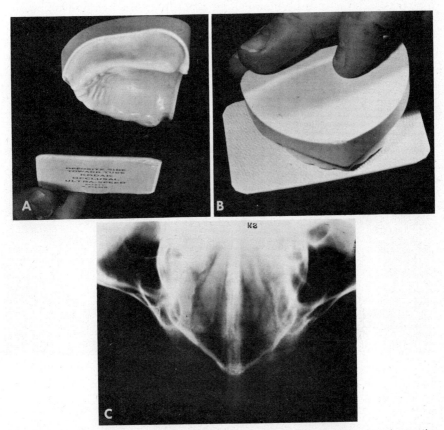

Figure 14–11 Maxillary occlusal exposure. *A* and *B*, The film is centered over the maxillary arch with the tube side of the film facing up. The film is placed breadthwise whenever possible. The patient retains the film in position by closing on it or by using thumb pressure against the ridges. *C*, Resultant radiograph.

should be made to bisect the angle formed by the ridge and film, although the vertical angulation may be as much as +55 to +65 degrees.

A truer image of the ridge may be obtained if the radiograph is taken with the film in an intraoral film holder. Although the image is better because the film and ridge are more nearly parallel, it is not always possible to use film holders, owing to anatomical restrictions such as those encountered in patients with low palates or small ridges.

When a film holder is employed, either a short cone or a long cone may be used, the unit being adjusted according to which one is chosen. No matter which is used, the vertical angulation is determined as in the bisection of the angle technique, but the angulation is less severe. In some cases the central ray may be almost perpendicular to the film, as in the long cone technique. Gauze or cotton rolls can be used on the biting surface of the film holder for the patient's comfort.

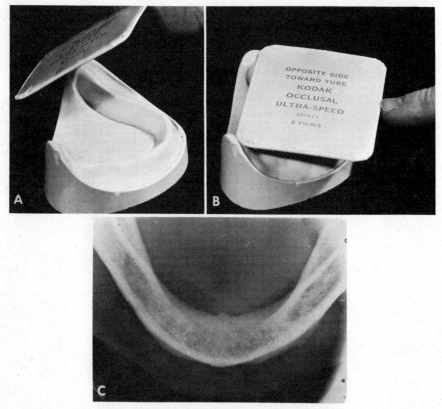

Figure 14–12 Mandibular occlusal exposure. *A* and *B*, The film is centered over the mandibular arch (on top of the tongue) with the tube side facing the mandibular arch. The film is placed breadthwise whenever possible. The patient retains the film in position by closing on it or by pressing down on the film with the index fingers. *C*, Resultant radiograph.

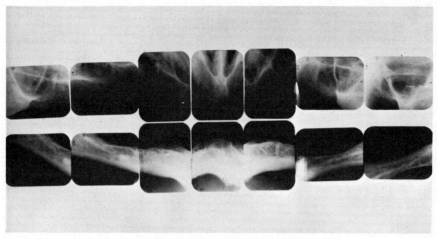

Figure 14–13   A mounted full series of exposed x-ray films of an edentulous patient.

An excellent supplemental film to the periapical series would be a maxillary and mandibular occlusal view. The procedure is the same as that described in Chapter 8 (Figs. 14–11 and 14–12).

A mounted full series of radiographs of an edentulous patient is shown in Figure 14–13.

REMINDERS

1. Know why you expose films of edentulous areas.
2. When exposing films of the periapical regions, the film tends to lie more nearly horizontally than in dentulous patients; therefore, some increase in vertical angulation is necessary.
3. Use the same horizontal angulations as those used for dentulous patients.
4. Note in the photographs how much of the film extends above or below the ridge, then place film accurately.

15

THE TEMPOROMANDIBULAR JOINT

No one can make you feel inferior without your consent.

Eleanor Roosevelt

The temporomandibular joint is the junction where the condyle of the mandible joins with the temporal bone of the skull (Fig. 15–1). The opening, closing, and lateral movements of the mandible are guided and supported by the bones and muscles of this joint. The T.M. joint, as it is commonly called, also contains ligaments strategically placed to prevent extreme movements of the mandible, such as opening too far. When the mouth is closed, the head of the condyle fits into the part of the temporal bone known as the glenoid fossa (Fig. 15–2). As the mouth opens, the head of the condyle slides forward to another area of the temporal bone, the articular eminence. The meniscus, a fibrocarti-

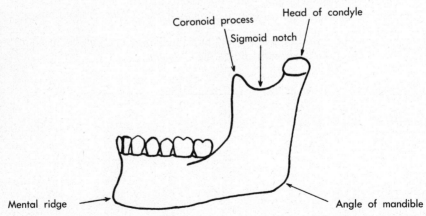

Figure 15-1 Diagram of the mandible showing the head of the condyle and other important landmarks of the mandible.

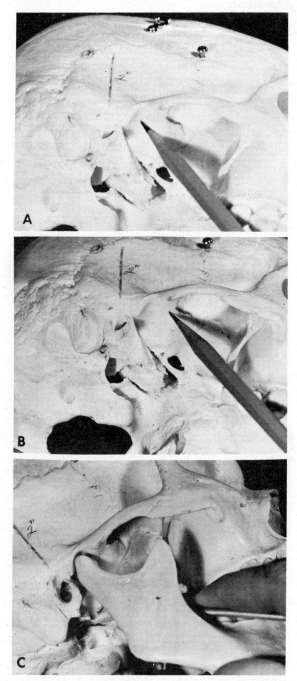

Figure 15–2 *A*, The tip of the pointer is in the center of the glenoid fossa. *B*, The tip of the pointer is on the articular eminence. *C*, Photograph of the T.M. joint showing the head of the condyle in its normal relation to the glenoid fossa.

laginous disk, separates the condyle from the glenoid fossa. It appears as a radiolucent space on a radiograph.

When there is a T.M. joint disturbance it is usually a manifestation of improper occlusion of the teeth. Other possible causes of T.M. joint disturbances are degeneration of bony structures, calcium deposits, tumors, infections, and arthritic conditions. The patient usually complains of pain in the area of the joint or the ear. The pain may be occasional or constant; it can occur on one or both sides; it may extend up into the head and down through the neck. A satisfactory diagnosis can be made only by a clinical examination in conjunction with radiographs of the joint. The radiographs will show the position of the condyle in the glenoid fossa of the temporal bone and, when the mouth is open, the relation of the condyle to the articular eminence (Fig. 15–3). A good

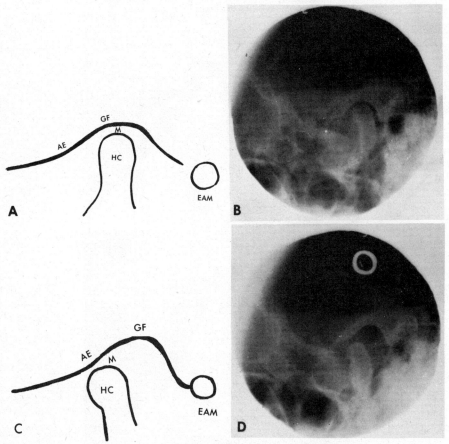

Figure 15–3 *A* and *B*, Diagram and radiograph of the T.M. joint with the patient's mouth closed and teeth in occlusion. *C* and *D*, Diagram and radiograph of the T.M. joint with the patient's mouth opened wide. (The "O" in the radiograph signifies the open position.) HC = Head of the condyle; M = meniscus; AE = articular eminence; GF = glenoid fossa; EAM = external auditory meatus.

set of radiographs will also show the effects of those pathologic conditions previously mentioned.

Treatment of these disturbances requires careful study of the radiographs. Finding the exact position of the condyle requires that the joint be viewed in at least two positions. The first radiograph should show the joint as it is when the patient's mouth is closed with the teeth in natural, habitual occlusion. The second view should be taken when the mouth is open as wide as possible. Some dentists like to have a third radiograph with the mandible in "rest" position. In this position the teeth are normally slightly apart and the muscles controlling mandibular movement are in a relaxed state.

During the course of treatment it is usually necessary to take at least one more series of radiographs at a later date for purposes of comparison. For this reason strict adherence to the procedure is necessary. The central ray must be directed through the joint at exactly the same angle, and the patient must assume the same position each time. This assures that the radiographs are duplicated correctly and that the movement of the condyle within the glenoid fossa and onto the articular eminence, which usually changes as the result of treatment, can be accurately noted.

The T.M. joint is exposed from the opposite side of the head. Therefore the x-ray beam must pass through the skull before it reaches the joint being exposed. In order to avoid as much superimposition of the other bony structures as possible, the central ray must pass through the joint from the most advantageous angle. According to Shore,* the superior surface of the condylar head and the inclination of the glenoid fossa are at an average angle of 25 degrees to the horizontal (Fig. 15–4). Therefore, by directing the central ray through the joint at a 25-degree angle, the radiograph will show the component parts of the joint from the most advantageous position.

A cassette with high-speed intensifying screens and high-speed film, such as Kodak's Blue Brand, is used in order to reduce exposure times. The screens will bring out the greatest amount of detail by reducing the amount of secondary radiation fogging the film. No more than six exposures should ever be taken at one sitting.

There are basically two techniques for taking T.M. joint exposures with dental x-ray units. The first one is the easier method for both you and the patient, because the radiograph is exposed while the patient is in the dental chair. The other technique differs from the first in that the patient's head must be positioned on a stationary cassette placed on a table top, rather than placing the cassette in position against the joint.

The radiographs obtained by either method, if correctly exposed,

---

*Shore, N. A: Occlusal Equilibration and Temporomandibular Joint Disfunction. Philadelphia, J. B. Lippincott Co., 1959.

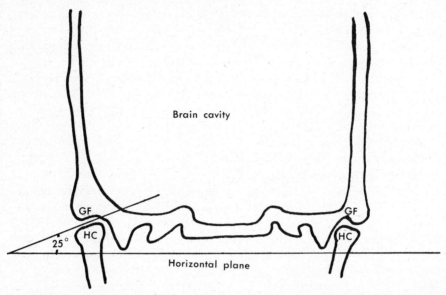

Figure 15–4   Diagrammatic sketch of the T.M. joint showing the 25-degree angle formed by the superior surface of the condylar head and the articular surface of the glenoid fossa. GF = Glenoid fossa; HC = head of the condyle.

will produce equally good results. Some authorities believe that the most accurate reading of the T.M. joint is obtained by the first procedure because the patient's head is held upright in a normal position. In the second method the head is tilted to one side and gravity tends to pull the mandible toward the side being exposed, resulting in an inaccurate registration of the joint.

Lead rubber or lead sheeting is used to cover the cassette so that more than one exposure can be made on each film. In the first procedure one half of the cassette front is covered for the first exposure; then the sheeting is moved to the opposite half for the second exposure (Fig. 15–5). A larger cassette is used for the second technique. A lead rubber sheet with a circular opening 2½ inches in diameter is placed on the cassette (Fig. 15–6). By changing the position of this sheet it is possible to expose, develop, and view four exposures on one film. Small wire letters, "R" or "L," should be taped to the cassette to indicate which joint is being exposed.

Technique I

A. Seat the patient comfortably in an upright position. The midline of the face should be perpendicular to the floor and the maxillary arch parallel to the floor.

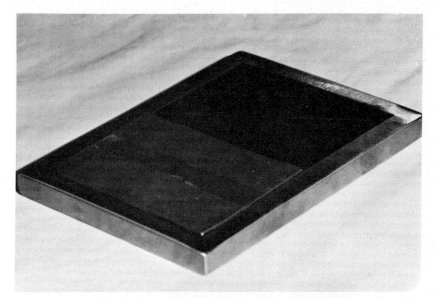

Figure 15–5   A 5 × 7 cassette with the lead sheeting covering one half of the surface.

B. A 5× 7 cassette with high-speed intensifying screens is used. Lead sheeting covers first one half, then the opposite half, during the exposures. One half is used to expose the joint with the teeth in occlusion and the other half with the mouth wide open. Center the un-

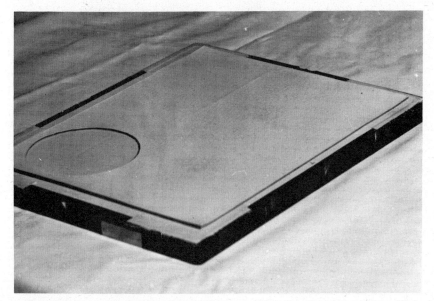

Figure 15–6   An 8 × 10 cassette with the lead rubber sheeting, from which a 2½ inch circle has been cut, covering the surface.

covered half of the cassette over the T.M. joint to be exposed. The midline of the face and the cassette should be parallel to one another (Fig. 15–7).

C. The cone is removed from the tube head to obtain a shortened target-film distance. By shortening this distance, the shadows of the intervening bony structures become so enlarged that they tend to become less obvious when viewing the image of the joint itself. The total filtration of the unit should equal 2.25 millimeters of aluminum, which is considered normal for modern dental units.* This amount of filtration filters out more of the less penetrating rays, a necessity because of the intensity of the x-rays at such a close position to the head.

---

*Richards, A. G., et al.: X-ray protection in the dental office. J.A.D.A., 56:514, 1958.
Wuehrmann, A. H.: Radiation Protection and Dentistry. St. Louis, C. V. Mosby Co., 1960.

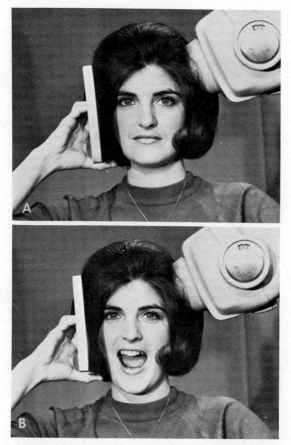

Figure 15–7 The correct position of the patient, cassette, and tube head for (A) the closed position and (B) the open position.

The central ray is projected toward the T.M. joint being exposed at an oblique angle of 25 degrees from a point 2 inches above the opposite external auditory meatus (outer opening of the ear) (Fig. 15–8). This is to avoid superimposition of one T.M. joint over the other (Fig. 15–9). A minimum of two exposures should be made of each joint, one with the teeth closed in normal occlusion and the other with the mouth open wide.

The exposure time with the unit operating on 65 KVP and 10 MA is approximately 1½ to 2½ seconds. The time varies depending upon the size of the patient and the density of the bone. If the developed film is too dark, decrease the exposure time; if it is too light, increase the time for subsequent exposures of the patient.

Technique II—Oblique Transcranial Projection

The advantage of this technique is that the procedure, i.e., the positioning of the head and cassette and the angling of the central rays, is so exact that accurate duplicating radiographs can easily be produced.

A. Place an 8 × 10 cassette, with lead sheeting in place, on top of a bench or table. Use a 25-degree angle board or prop the upper edge of

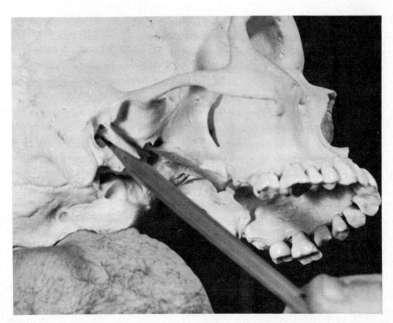

Figure 15–8 The pointer is locating a small round opening into the skull. This is the external auditory meatus and it is immediately posterior to the glenoid fossa. On the radiograph this structure appears as a round radiolucent landmark.

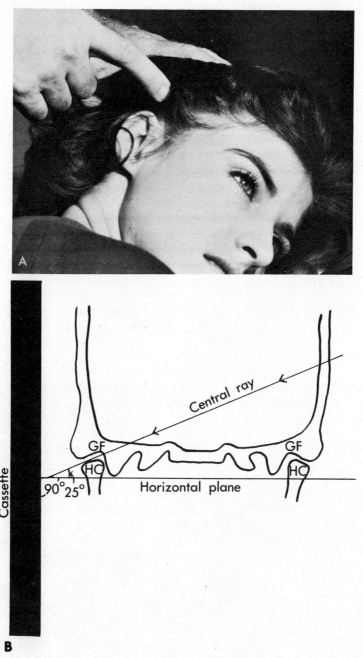

Figure 15–9 *A*, The point of entrance of the central ray for radiographs of the opposite T.M. joint. *B*, Diagram of the position of the cassette in relation to the T.M. joint being exposed for Technique I.

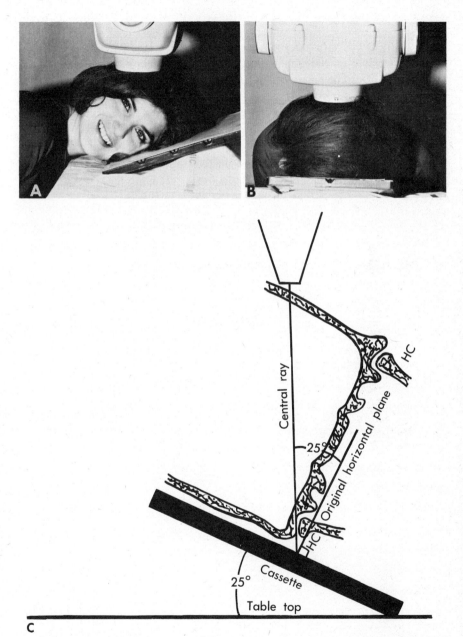

Figure 15–10   Oblique transcranial projection. *A* and *B,* The correct position of the patient, cassette, and tube head for this technique. *C,* Diagram of the position of the cassette in relation to the T.M. joint being exposed.

the cassette so that it makes an angle of 25 degrees with the horizontal table top.

B. Seat the patient in a chair. Be certain not to place his legs under the table, thus avoiding direct exposure of reproductive organs to the central ray. Place his head on the cassette with the T.M. joint to be exposed centered over the circular opening. Only the area of the temple should come in contact with the cassette.

C. The cone tip is removed as in Technique I. The central ray is projected from a point 2 inches above the external auditory meatus. The angle of the central ray should be perpendicular (90 degrees) to the table top. For an x-ray unit operating on 65 KVP and 10 MA the approximate exposure time is $1\frac{1}{2}$ to $2\frac{1}{2}$ seconds, as in Technique I.

Take four exposures, as in the previous procedure. Put the open and closed views of this joint on one half of the film. To expose the other joint, reverse the lead sheet on the cassette so that the other half of the film can be exposed; face the patient in the opposite direction (Fig. 15–10).

REMINDERS

1. Correct positioning of the patient's head and the cone tip are of utmost importance.
2. Know why the 25-degree vertical angle to the horizontal plane is used (Fig. 13–4).
3. Mark "R" or "L" to indicate which side is being exposed.
4. For future T. M. joint exposures, the same head and cone tip placement as the original must be used if correct comparisons are to be made.

16

THE FIVE MOST COMMON ERRORS IN TECHNIQUE

Real joy comes not from ease or riches or from the praise of men, but from doing something worthwhile.

Grenfell

Even though the techniques for the different radiographic procedures are followed with great attention to detail, you will find especially in the learning stages that an occasional radiograph will not be satisfactory. The errors most frequently encountered and the methods for their correction are listed here.

Elongation. Elongation is the most frequent error made by beginners. When the image of the tooth, as seen on the x-ray film, is longer than the tooth itself, it is called elongation. This occurs because of insufficient vertical angulation of the tube head. In the maxillary arch elongation is a result of not increasing the angulation enough to bisect the angle. For example, if +45 degrees is necessary for correctly exposing a certain tooth and the angle used is only +30 degrees, the resultant image will be too long. In the mandibular arch elongation occurs when the minus vertical angulation is not increased sufficiently. A vertical angulation of −15 degrees will cause elongation when the angulation should have been −30 degrees for bisection of the angle (Fig. 16–1).

Foreshortening. Foreshortening is the opposite of elongation. The image of the tooth on the x-ray film is shorter than the actual tooth, and this is caused by too much vertical angulation. If a vertical angulation of +45 degrees is necessary for correct bisection and the angulation is set at +55 degrees, foreshortening occurs (Fig. 16–2).

Horizontal Overlap. Horizontal overlap is the superimposition of the interproximal surfaces of adjacent teeth. This occurs when the cen-

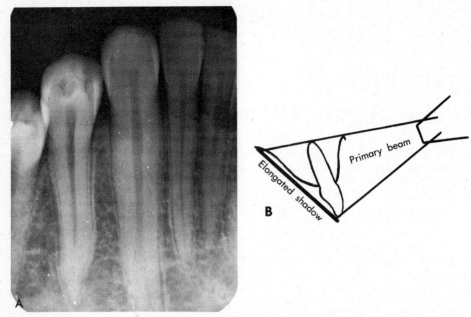

Figure 16–1 *A,* Radiograph exhibiting elongated images of the teeth. *B,* Diagrammatic sketch showing how elongation occurs.

tral rays are not directed through the contact points parallel to the interproximal surfaces (Fig. 16–3).

Cone Cutting.   Cone cutting or coning off is the error made when a film has been only partially exposed. This occurs when the x-ray

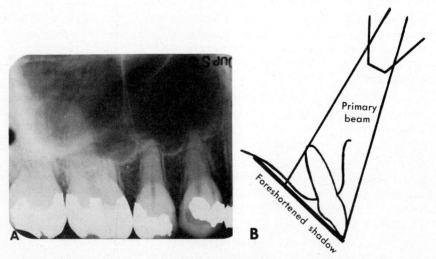

Figure 16–2 *A,* Radiograph exhibiting foreshortened images of the teeth. *B,* Diagrammatic sketch showing how foreshortening occurs.

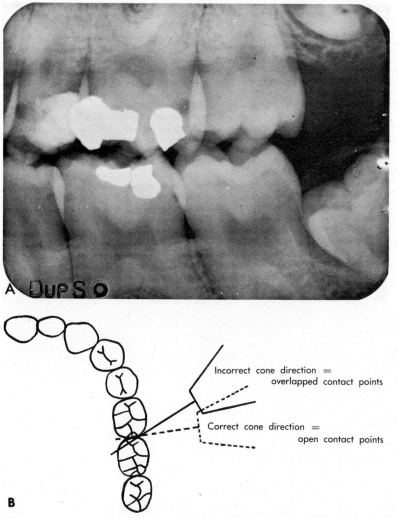

Figure 16-3 *A,* Radiograph exhibiting horizontal overlapping of the teeth. *B,* Diagrammatic sketch showing improper horizontal angulation resulting in superimposed proximal surfaces of the teeth (horizontal overlap).

beam is not directed to the center of the film, thereby leaving a portion of the film unexposed. The unexposed area will be clear on the processed film (Fig. 16–4).

Excessive Bending. Excessive bending of the film is most frequently found in exposures of the cuspid regions. When this occurs, that portion of the film which was bent will have an image similar to an elongated image. However, only the roots of the teeth appear distorted while the crowns remain relatively true in dimension, whereas an

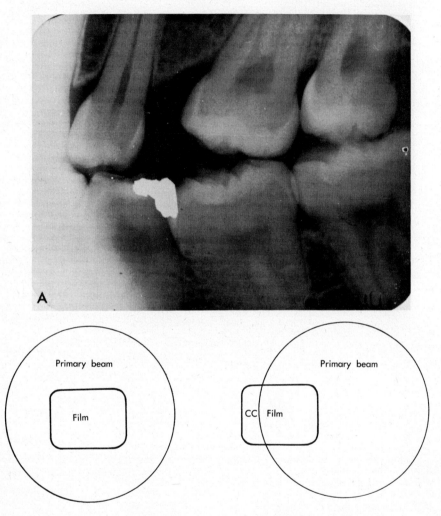

Primary beam directed to center of film insuring adequate exposure of entire film.

Primary beam directed away from center of film resulting in inadequate exposure of film known as cone cutting (cc).

Figure 16–4 *A,* Radiograph exhibiting unexposed clear area caused by cone cutting. *B,* Diagrammatic sketches showing how cone cutting occurs.

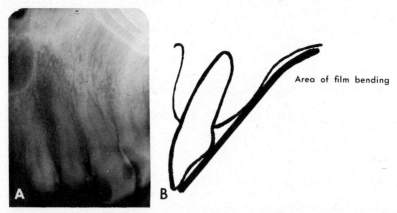

Figure 16–5 *A,* Radiograph exhibiting distorted area of film caused by excessive bending. *B,* Diagrammatic sketch showing how excessive bending occurs.

elongated image is distorted in all areas. The cause of excessive bending is improper finger pressure when holding the film in place. By applying the retentive finger pressure on the film at the crown-gingival junction of the teeth being exposed, the film should remain fairly straight throughout its entire length, thus eliminating the excessive bending. In Figure 16–5 *A,* the upper right corner of the film was bent to such a degree that the x-rays were parallel to the film and did not sufficiently expose it in that area.

REMINDERS

1. To correct elongation, use more vertical angulation.
2. To correct foreshortening, use less vertical angulation.
3. To correct horizontal overlap, direct the central ray parallel to the interproximal surfaces of the teeth.
4. To correct cone cutting, aim the central ray to the center of the film.
5. Excessive film bending is usually caused by excessive finger pressure too high or too low on the film.

17

RECOGNIZING OTHER IMPERFECTIONS

I am a great believer in luck, and I find the harder I work the more I have of it.

Stephen Leacock

Occasionally the radiographs you take will not be perfect. The imperfections are usually caused by mistakes made during processing or by faulty techniques other than those discussed in Chapter 14. Following are some of these imperfections you may observe on a processed radiograph.

LIGHT IMAGE (Fig. 17-1)

A radiograph with a weak image (too light) may be caused by one or more of the following factors.

Underdevelopment. This results from removing the film from the developing solution before the time needed to complete the development process has elapsed. This premature removal does not allow enough time for all the silver halide crystals to be partially or completely reduced to black metallic silver. Underdevelopment also occurs if the developing solution is too weak or exhausted from overuse or contamination. In either case the radiographic image has the overall appearance of being too light and lacks density.

Cold Processing Solutions. A radiographic image identical to that just described will be the result if the solutions are too cold during the development procedure. A low temperature retards the developing and fixing reaction with the emulsion of the film. If the film is not left in the solutions for an extra length of time, the chemical reactions will not go to completion.

196

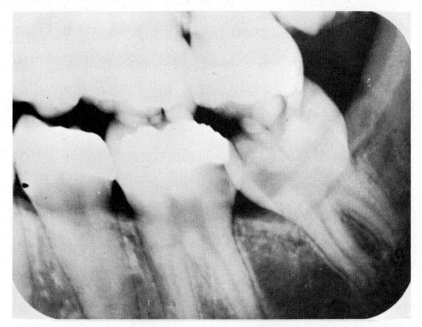

Figure 17–1 A light or weak image plus improper film placement for a bite-wing exposure.

Underexposure.   Underexposing the film also causes a light radiographic image. It is due to a lack of x-rays reaching the emulsion of the film. Either an inadequate amount of x-rays is generated from the tube, or most of those that are generated lack the ability to penetrate the dense tissues of the oral region and therefore do not reach the film. Be sure to firmly press the activating button and hold it until the unit shuts off automatically. This will ensure an adequate exposure time. Also be sure to doublecheck the dials on the x-ray cabinet to be certain the unit is operating at the required specifications. In Figure 15–1 you can see too much of the lower arch and not enough of the upper arch. This is a bite-wing exposure; when the patient closed on the bite-wing tab the cusps of the upper teeth engaged the superior edge of the film and pushed it down. An equal part of both arches should appear on a bite-wing radiograph.

DARK IMAGE (Fig. 17–2)

A radiograph with a dark image and too much density can be caused by conditions which are the opposite of those just listed.

If the dark image was caused by overdevelopment, check on the timing of the development process. If it was caused by processing solu-

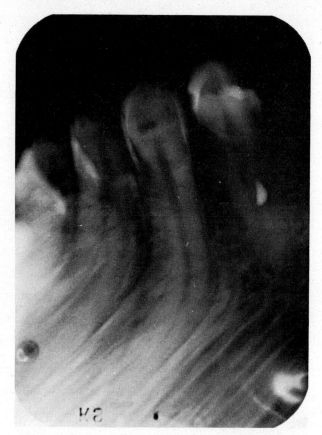

Figure 17–2 A dark image plus too much film bending.

tions that are too warm, be sure to control the temperature more closely during processing. Overexposure to x-rays can be avoided if the timer and dials on the x-ray cabinet are operating at the required specifications for the particular exposure you are taking. In Figure 17–2 the bony trabeculations near the crest of the ridge have been "burned out" as the result of overexposure. This radiograph also shows distortion in the lower half due to bending of the film.

Fogged Film (**Fig. 17–3**). The overall appearance of a fogged film is also dark, but it differs from the dark film just described because the images lack definition and appear as though they are being viewed through fog. Fogging is usually due to an excessive amount of light reaching the film from an improper dark room safe light, from light leaks around the dark room door, or from turning on a white light before the film is adequately fixed. An outdated film, even when exposed correctly, has a degree of fog imparted to it.

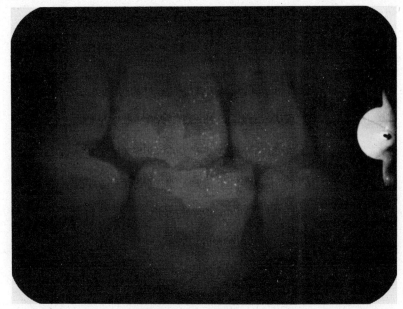

Figure 17–3 Fogged film.

BLANK OR BLACK FILM

Blank Film. A blank film usually results when no x-rays are generated in the tube during what you thought was the exposure time. If this is the case, the silver halide crystals did not become activated by any x-rays and all the unexposed crystals were removed in the fixing solution, resulting in a blank film. To prevent this from happening, make sure the unit is plugged into the electrical outlet securely and that it is functioning properly. Many dental offices have a central x-ray cabinet that will operate two or more x-ray units in separate operatories. If you are using this type of unit, be certain you have made the selection for the operatory in which you wish to x-ray the patient.

Another cause for a blank film may be processing solutions that are too warm. The emulsion will blister and dissolve from the film base, leaving a blank film. Maintain a constant check on the temperature of the solutions.

Black Film (**Fig. 17–4**). If a film is exposed to a white light or to daylight, even for an instant, the result will be a black film. Remember that the x-ray film emulsion is very sensitive to white light; you should be certain that there is no light leakage around the edge of the door. During the processing stage there should be absolutely no light in the dark room except that from the safe light. An improperly filtered safe light may severely blacken a film if the film is exposed to it long enough.

Figure 17–4 Black film.

PROCESSING ERRORS

White Streaks or Spots (**Fig. 17–5**).   If a developed film is stained with white spots or streaks, it is probably because the fixer solution came into contact with the film before it was routinely developed. These spots are white or lighter in appearance because the silver halide reduction to black metallic silver, which normally occurs in the developing solution, has been blocked by the fixer solution. Placing the film on a dark room table that has been splashed with fixing solution is the usual cause of such spots. Streaks are the result of the film clip being contaminated with fixer solution. When the film is placed on a contaminated clip, the solution rolls over the surface of the film. To protect against these faults, be sure that the table top on which the films are being stripped has been wiped clean and dry and that the film racks have been thoroughly washed and dried before being used for further development of film.

Black Streaks or Spots.   In Figure 17–6 there is a dark streak just left of the center of the radiograph. A drop of developer solution prematurely developed the film as it rolled over the surface of the emulsion. When the film was placed in the developer solution for normal development, the area where the drop prematurely contacted the film became overdeveloped, causing the dark streak. Again, a clean, dry table top and film racks will prevent this.

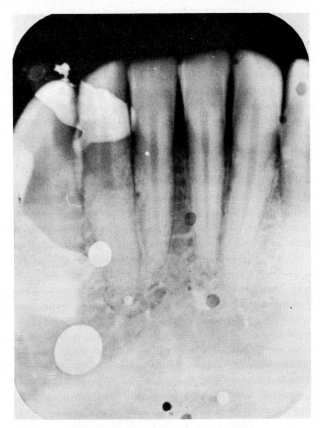

Figure 17–5   White streaks or spots.

Opaque Spots.   Opaque areas are caused by one film clinging to another or the side of the tank during the fixation process. This causes the film to retain the silver salts normally removed by the fixing solution, because the fixer didn't reach these areas. To prevent this, always agitate the films briefly when placing them in the solution.

Dark Brown or Gray Film.   A film that appears dark brown or gray has not been properly fixed. Either the film was not left in the fixer solution for the required length of time (the unexposed silver crystals are not removed), or the fixing solution is exhausted from age or overuse.

Brownish-Yellow Stain.   Insufficient rinsing after the film has been completely processed results in a brownish-yellow chemical stain remaining in the emulsion of the film.

Heavily Stained Film.   In Figure 17–7 a stripped film was placed on a table top contaminated with puddles of water or other chemical-containing liquids prior to being placed in the developer. This resulted in the film being permanently stained.

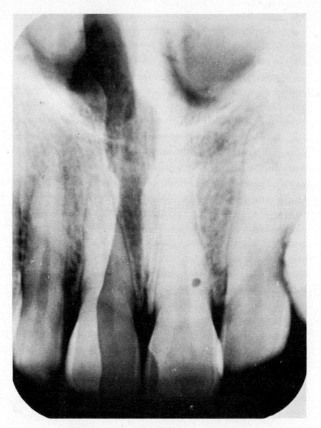

Figure 17–6 Black streaks or spots.

Scratched Film. Scratches such as those seen in Figure 17–8 are caused by laying the wet film on an unclean surface or by placing it against sharp or pointed objects (fingernails, film clips, and so on). The film emulsion is softened upon contact with any moisture; such film requires very careful handling until it is completely processed and dried.

Torn Film. When the film is removed from the packet too hastily, a torn film is usually the result. In Figure 17–9 the film was pulled from the packet before it was completely freed from the paper wrapping.

ERRORS IN TECHNIQUE

Reversed Film (**Fig. 17–10**). When the film is exposed with the wrong side facing the tube, the x-rays must pass through the lead foil backing. This backing prohibits some x-rays from reaching the film.

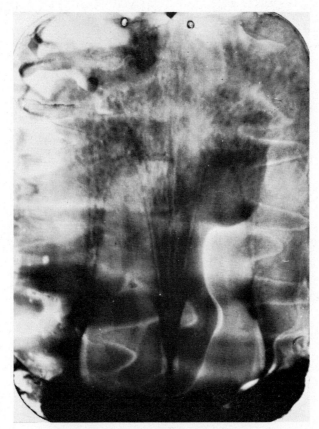

Figure 17-7   Heavily stained film.

The resultant images lack density, and the overall appearance is lighter and weaker than normal. You can also notice on the film a peculiar pattern of dark marks known as the "herringbone pattern." This is due to the embossed pattern on the lead foil backing. The images on this film are reversed in relation to the embossed dot.

Saliva Leak (**Fig. 17–11**).   If the film is bent too sharply when you attempt to make it conform to the curvature of the mouth, the seal around the edge of the packet may break. This allows saliva to leak into the film. When it contacts the film emulsion, it causes the surrounding black envelope to adhere to the film. Later, when the film is stripped, the black paper envelope remains stuck to the film in these areas.

Double Exposure.   A double exposure is the result when an exposed film is inadvertently placed back into the mouth and re-exposed. In Figure 17–12 the anterior teeth are superimposed over the posterior teeth. Because the film was exposed twice it has an overall appearance of being too dark.

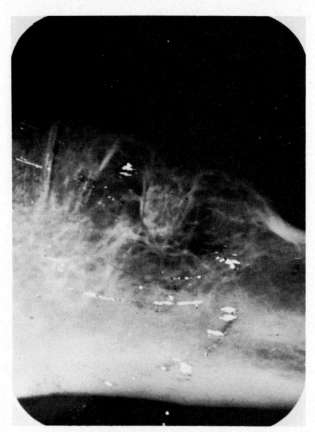

Figure 17-8 Scratched film.

Incorrect Film Placement. In Figure 17–13 the root apices of the second molar are cut off at the top of the radiograph. This error was caused by not placing the inferior edge of the film parallel to the occlusal plane of the teeth. The posterior portion of the film was placed too low in relation to the teeth.

Double Image (**Fig. 17–14**). A double image is caused when the film is moved slightly during the exposure and then held firmly in the new position during the remainder of the exposure. The image is doubled or has a shadowy appearance. Always instruct the patient to hold the film securely in the exact position you have placed it. The patient should let you know if the film moves during the exposure. If this is a problem with a particular patient you might use one of the many film holders on the market to hold the film in position. Once the film is in position, instruct the patient to bite on the holder to maintain the film position.

Blurred Image (**Fig. 17–15**). A blurred image is usually caused when the tube head moves slightly back and forth during the exposure

Text continued on page 209

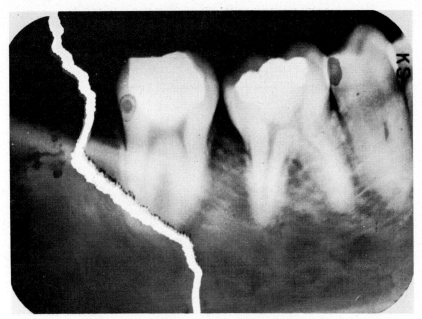

Figure 17–9   Torn film.

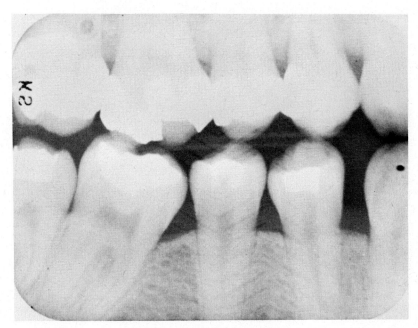

Figure 17–10   Reversed film.

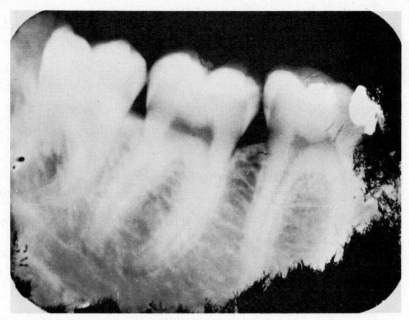

Figure 17–11 Saliva leak.

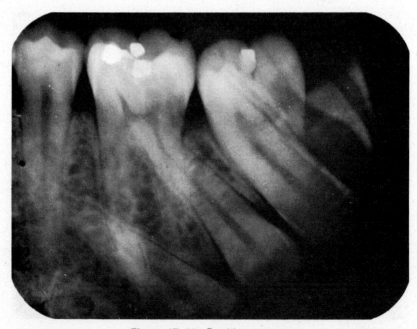

Figure 17–12 Double exposure.

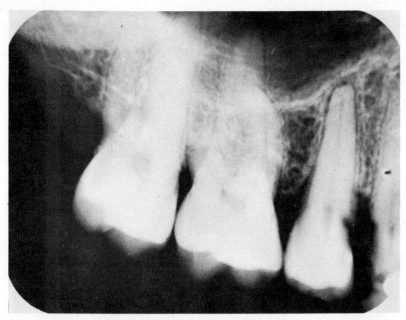

Figure 17–13 Incorrect film placement.

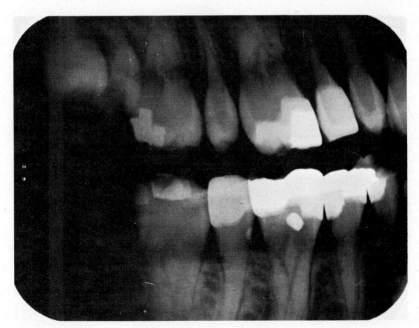

Figure 17–14 Double image.

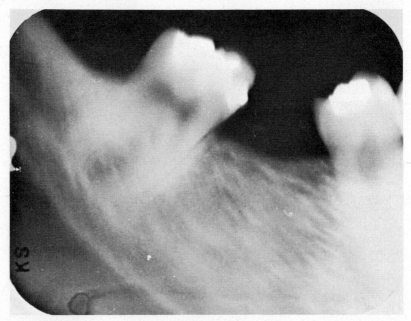

Figure 17–15 Blurred image.

of the film. However, movement of the patient's head, as well as film slippage during the exposure, will tend to blur the image.

Superimposed Images.   Failure to remove any partial or complete denture will result in superimposition of these structures over the areas exposed. In Figure 17–16A the artificial teeth can be seen in the lower portion of the radiograph, although the x-rays were able to penetrate the acrylic portion of the denture. The bone tissue looks fairly clear and well defined, but it would appear clearer had the denture been removed. In Figure 17–16B the metal framework of a partial denture can be seen. The x-rays were not capable of penetrating the metal and therefore left the radiograph white in this area.

Occasionally a finger will be superimposed over the teeth. This happens when the patient's fingers lie in the path of the central rays during the exposure (Fig. 17–17). When the patient holds the film in place with his thumb or index finger, the remaining fingers of the hand must be tightly clenched into a fist or straightened out away from the x-

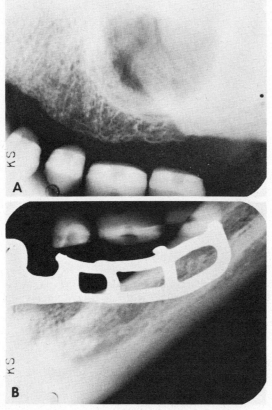

Figure 17–16 *A,* Upper denture left in the mouth during the exposure. *B,* Lower partial denture left in the mouth during the exposure.

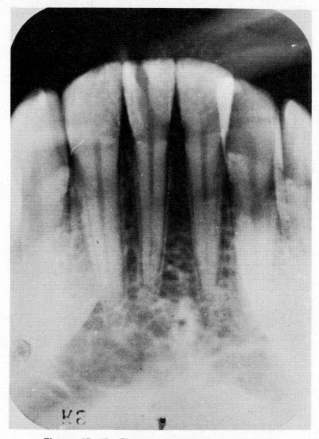

Figure 17–17 Finger superimposed over teeth.

ray beam. If these fingers are allowed to relax, they will usually be in the path of the x-ray beam.

REMINDERS

1. Always check the operation of the unit at the beginning of each day.
2. Make sure the door to the dark room is closed tightly before stripping the film.
3. Before laying stripped film down on the table top, be certain the surface is clean and dry.
4. Other than solution, do not allow anything to touch the film emulsion before it is dry.
5. To prevent double exposure, clip film to the film rack immediately following its exposure.
6. Remove partials or removable bridges before radiographing your patient.

18

MAKING USE OF THE RADIOGRAPH

Our imagination is the only limit to what we can hope to have in the future.

Charles Kettering

Although the dental hygienist or assistant is not permitted to diagnose from a radiograph, the author feels that you should be cognizant of the information revealed by a radiographic examination. If you have not already, you will in the future hear the dentist say such things as "this appears to be a cyst," "the root of the tooth shows a fracture line," "look at this interproximal bone loss," and so forth. Have you ever wondered how these and many other findings appear on the radiograph?

When a patient complains of swelling or of pain in a certain area, the dentist will usually make a preliminary clinical examination in order to find the causative factor. If necessary information is not revealed, he may request that you x-ray the area to reinforce his clinical findings. Accurate film placement and correct angulations are most important when studying radiographs for pathology. The radiographs in this chapter exhibit some of the most frequently observed lesions that cause the patient to seek relief through treatment.

CARIES

Dental caries are defects in the enamel due to decalcification. X-rays readily penetrate these areas of decalcified enamel, and the caries therefore have a radiolucent appearance when seen on the radiograph. Once the carious lesion penetrates the outer enamel covering of the crown, it rapidly enlarges in size because of the decreased density of the dentin in comparison with the enamel.

Several carious lesions can be seen in the primary teeth in Figure 18–1 and in several permanent teeth in Figure 18–2. In Figure 18–3, the mandibular second molar has been extracted. The third molar has

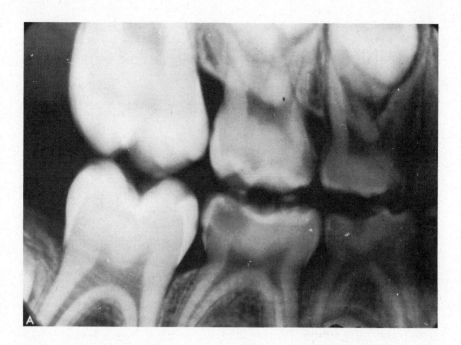

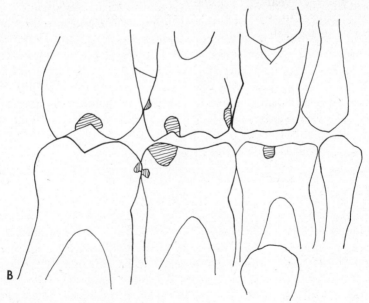

Figure 18–1 *A*, Carious lesions in primary molars and first permanent molars. *B*, Shaded areas denote carious lesions in *A*.

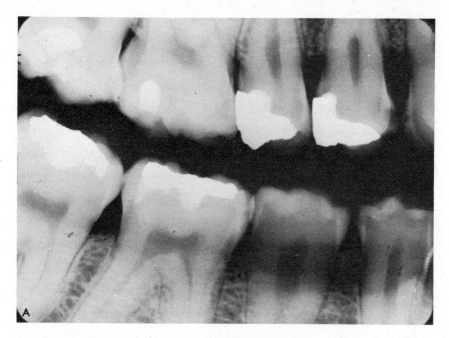

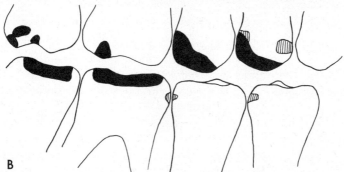

Figure 18-2 *A*, Carious lesions in permanent teeth. *B*, Lined areas denote carious lesions in *A*. Blackened areas denote metallic fillings.

tilted into the second molar space and has become locked under the crown of the first molar. Owing to the difficulty of keeping this area clean, a carious lesion can be observed as a radiolucent area expanding outward from the contact point of the third molar.

ACUTE AND CHRONIC PERIAPICAL ABSCESSES

These lesions begin to form when the dental pulp of the affected tooth is infected with bacteria, usually from a carious lesion. A blow to

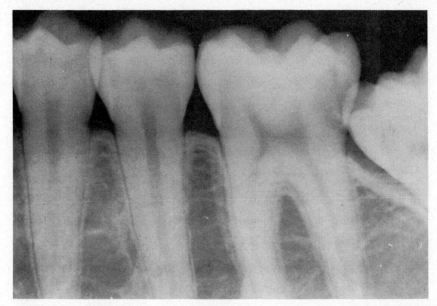

Figure 18–3 Third molar causing a carious lesion to form in the second molar.

a tooth, if severe enough, will also cause the pulp to degenerate, leading to an abscess formation. Before the effects of an abscess can be seen on a radiograph, the toxic material must pass through the pulp canal to the apical foramen. Once it reaches the apex of the tooth, decalcification takes place in the bony tissue surrounding the apex. Approximately one third of the bone calcium must be lost before radiographic evidence of an abscess can be demonstrated. The longer the abscess has a chance to develop, the darker it will appear on the radiograph.

In observing Figure 18–4A, an area of radiolucency appears at the apical region of the mandibular second molar. The lamina dura surrounding the mesial root apex is obliterated. This is highly indicative of abscess formation. Note the deep cavity preparation.

In Figure 18–4B, there is an area of developing radiolucency at the apex of the maxillary lateral incisor. An apical thickening of the periodontal membrane space with obliteration of the lamina dura can be seen. The radiolucent area is poorly circumscribed, which indicates an acute type of abscess. The same condition appears on the central incisor. Note also the large carious lesions on the mesial surfaces of the involved teeth.

In Figure 18–4C, a faint area of radiolucency surrounds the apical area of the maxillary lateral incisor. There is thickening of the periodontal membrane space, plus a loss in continuity of the lamina dura surrounding the apex. The deep carious lesion at the mesial surface of

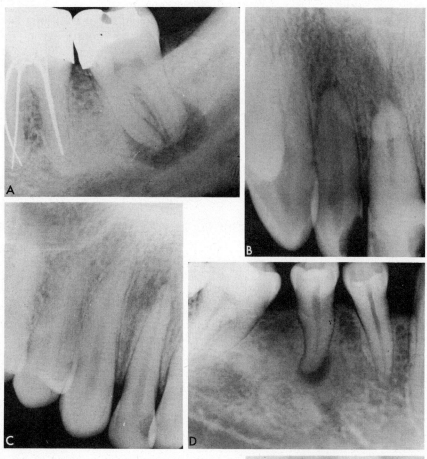

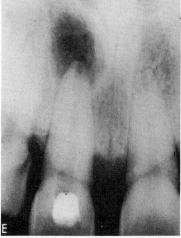

Figure 18–4 Apical abscess of mandibular second molar (*A*), maxillary lateral incisor (*B*), maxillary lateral incisor (*C*), mandibular second bicuspid (*D*), and maxillary central incisor (*E*).

the lateral incisor appears to extend to involve the pulp. Because of its diffuse outline, the lesion would indicate an acute abscess.

An area of radiolucency surrounds the apex of the mandibular second bicuspid in Figure 18–4D. There is gross discontinuity of the periodontal membrane space and the lamina dura. The lesion is identified by a dark radiolucency, which indicates chronic abscess formation. The mental foramen is seen in this area as a faint radiolucency just below the abscess. An identical appearing lesion is seen at the apex of the right central incisor in Figure 18–4E. The prominent radiolucency with a fairly well defined border suggests that the lesion has been present for quite some time. This chronic lesion is in contrast to the diffuse border and not so radiolucent lesion seen in the acute abscess formation.

PERIAPICAL CYSTS

An abscessed tooth, if allowed to remain untreated, may develop a root end cyst. The cyst itself is a sac containing fluid and causes a round or ovoid cavity of varying size to form in the bone. Although the cyst cannot with certainty be distinguished from an abscess when viewing a radiograph, there is one feature which suggests that the lesion is a cyst—the well-defined outline of cortical bone. Because the lesion is slow-growing in nature, there is a tendency for the body defenses to wall off the diseased area by forming this border of dense cortical bone.

In these radiographs, a radiolucent image is seen over the maxillary first bicuspid (Fig. 18–5A) as well as the maxillary second bicuspid (Fig. 18–5B). Both of these lesions are surrounded by a thin white outline of cortical bone that suggests the lesions to be cysts.

BONE SCLEROSIS (OSTEOSCLEROSIS, CONDENSING OSTEITIS)

Excessively radiopaque or light areas of bone represent an increase in the calcification of the bone involved. As we saw earlier, the area of an abscess appears dark owing to the x-rays' easy penetration of the lesion. The lesser the amount of calcium in the bone, the lesser the number of x-rays absorbed by the bone, thus allowing more x-rays to penetrate to the film and give a darker appearance to the area on the radiograph. In the case of sclerotic bone, just the opposite is true. The greater the calcification, the lighter or more opaque the bone image will appear.

There are two basic causes for this type of bone formation. One is repair of a diseased area that has been resolved, such as a former abscess. Just as nature overresponds to the repair of a broken arm or leg with new, very dense bone, so she responds to the repair of bone sur-

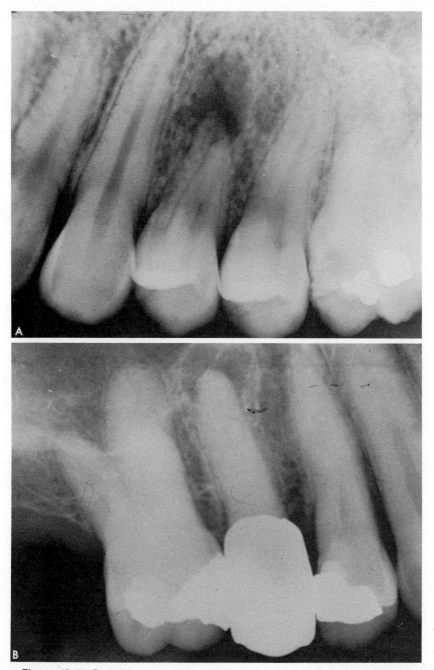

Figure 18–5 Probable cystic lesion at root apex of first bicuspid (*A*) and second bicuspid (*B*).

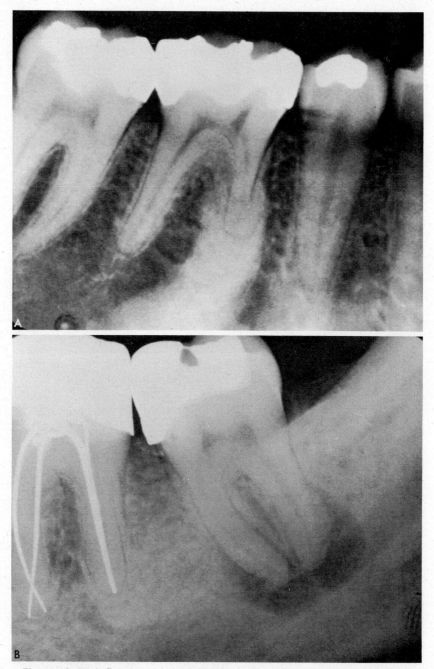

Figure 18–6 *A,* Dense area of sclerotic bone surrounds root of the infected mandibular first molar. *B,* Diffuse area of sclerotic bone surrounds root of the mandibular second molar.

Illustration continued on opposite page

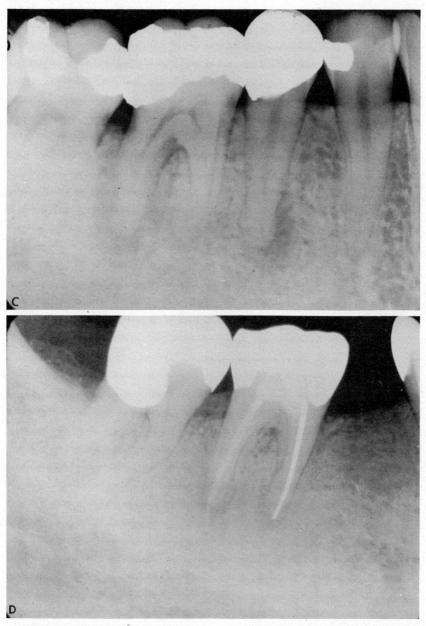

Figure 18–6 *Continued.*   *C,* Diffuse area of sclerotic bone over the posterior area of the mandible. *D,* Sclerotic bone surrounds endodontically treated mandibular first molar.

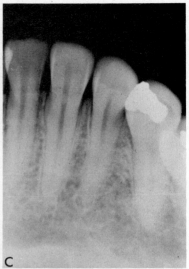

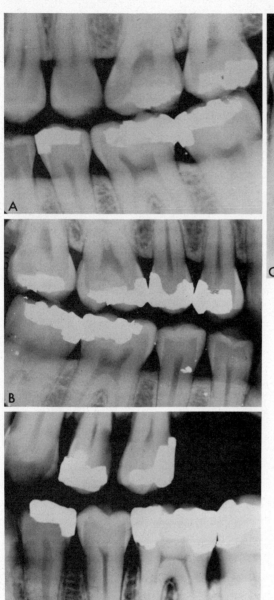

Figure 18–7 *A, B,* and *C,* Normal, healthy support bone. Height of alveolar crest is located at crown-root junction. *D,* Beginning destruction of alveolar bone crest. Bone recession indicates periodontitis is present.

Illustration continued on opposite page

rounding the teeth with very dense bone. The other reason sclerotic bone may be formed is in an attempt to wall off inflammation or spreading infection. The dense bone becomes a line of resistance.

In Figure 18–6*A,* the mesial root of the mandibular first molar is involved in an area of localized sclerotic bone. The radiopaque area of abnormally dense bone has actually stimulated the resorption of the

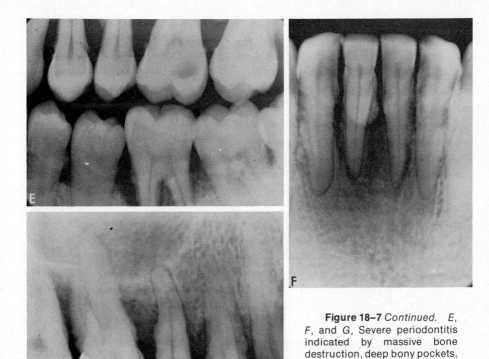

Figure 18–7 *Continued.* E, F, and G, Severe periodontitis indicated by massive bone destruction, deep bony pockets, and large deposits of calculus.

apical third of the root. The mandibular second molar in Figure 18–6*B* has an apical infection surrounded by diffuse sclerotic bone. Figure 18–6*C* reveals that much of the posterior region of the mandible is involved with a diffuse area of sclerotic bone. Infections at the root apices of the first molar and the second bicuspid are probably the stimulating factors in this dense bone formation. In Figure 18–6*D*, the diffuse area of sclerotic bone is probably due to the apical involvement of the mandibular first molar. Notice that the tooth has been treated endodontically, with the root canals being filled. If this treatment is successful, the sclerotic bone may revert back to normal bone over a period of time.

PERIODONTAL DISEASE

Periodontal disease affects the supporting structures of the teeth, such as the periodontal ligament which occupies the periodontal membrane space, the supporting alveolar bone, and the gingiva. Now that more teeth are being saved, there is a corresponding rise in periodontal disease.

The first stage of periodontal disease is gingivitis, which is inflammation confined to the gingiva. This is usually brought on by a buildup of calculus at the gingival margins of the teeth. Overhanging restorations and a lack of good oral hygiene are causative factors also.

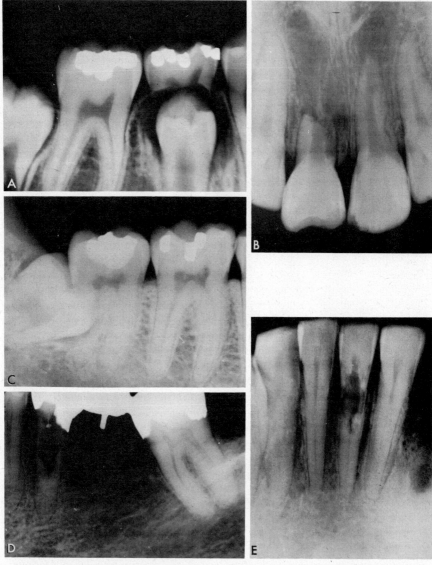

Figure 18–8 *A*, Resorption of primary molar ahead of erupting permanent bicuspid. *B*, Resorption of root of the maxillary central incisor. *C*, Impacted mandibular third molar causing resorption of the adjacent second molar. *D*, Internal resorption of the mandibular second bicuspid. *E*, Internal resorption of the mandibular central incisor.

Because gingivitis involves the gingiva, which is soft tissue, the radiograph will appear normal. The alveolar bone crest will be positioned at, or close to, the crown-root junction. The periodontal membrane space and cortical bone appear normal as they surround the root of the tooth (Figs. 18–7A, 18–7B, and 18–7C).

If the patient does not seek treatment for gingivitis, the disease process will expand to involve the supporting bone and the periodontal membrane. The first radiographic signs are a destruction of the cortical crest and widening of the periodontal membrane space at the coronal third of the root (Fig. 18–7D). As the disease progresses, the support bone will be continually destroyed by the infection, gross calculus deposits will form subgingivally, and the teeth may become loose and exfoliate (Figs. 18–7E, 18–7F, and 18–7G).

RESORPTION OF TOOTH STRUCTURE

Prior to being shed, the roots of primary teeth undergo resorption ahead of the erupting permanent teeth. This is expected and considered normal, as in Figure 18–8A. There may be instances in which the permanent tooth erupts before the primary root resorbs completely, leaving a primary root fragment entrapped in alveolar bone.

Many times you will see an isolated tooth, such as a maxillary cen-

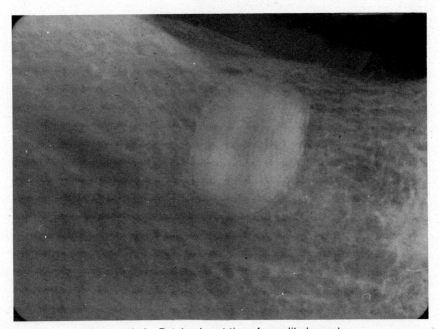

Figure 18–9   Retained root tips of mandibular molar.

tral incisor, in which the root has undergone resorption. This type of resorption is usually caused by injury to the tooth from a fall or a blow (Fig. 18–8B). Such injuries are one of the main causes of external resorption, others being an orthodontic appliance that has been worn for a time, an impacted tooth applying pressure to an adjacent tooth and subsequently causing its resorption (Fig. 18–8C), and formation of sclerotic bone that impinges on a root (Fig. 18–6A).

Another type of resorptive process frequently seen is internal resorption that takes place from the interior part of the tooth. There is resorption from the wall of the pulp chamber extending into dentin (Figs. 18–8D and 18–8E). This type can be found in either the root or the crown of the tooth. The exact cause of the interior resorptive process is not known. Systemic disease, inflammation of the pulp tissue, and trauma are possible causes.

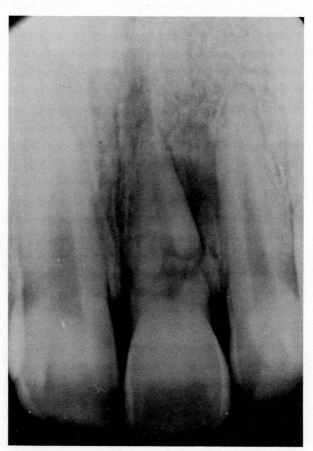

Figure 18–10 Root fracture of maxillary left central incisor.

ROOT TIPS RETAINED IN ALVEOLAR BONE

During the extraction of a tooth there is always a possibility that some part of the root may remain in the alveolar bone. The radiographic appearance of a retained root tip may resemble an area of sclerotic bone; however, a root tip will usually exhibit a nerve canal and a periodontal ligament space surrounding the radiopacity (Fig. 18–9).

ROOT FRACTURE

This is not an uncommon injury and is especially prevalent in children during the summer months. A fall at the swimming pool or a blow to the mouth while playing ball are frequent causes of root frac-

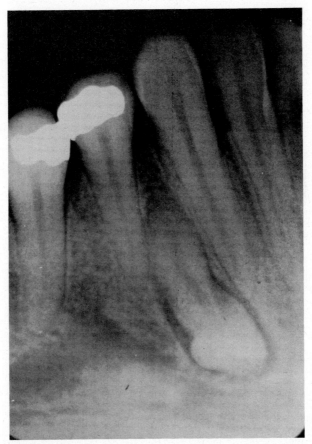

Figure 18–11 Mandibular cuspid area in which an inverted malformed supernumerary tooth can be seen.

tures. Though a fracture of the crown portion of the tooth can be seen clinically, a radiograph is necessary to discern a root fracture. Since the fracture is a separation of two radiopaque segments, you will observe a dark line through the root at the area of the fracture (Fig. 18–10).

SUPERNUMERARY TEETH

Some patients have one or more teeth in excess of the normal number. These "extra" teeth are known as supernumerary teeth. They are most frequently found in the maxillary incisor region, the next highest incidence being in the mandibular bicuspid region (Fig. 18–11). At times a fourth molar may be seen, but it is generally half the size or less than that of the other molars. A supernumerary tooth is usually impacted in bone and may prevent the eruption of a permanent tooth.

19

ANATOMICAL LANDMARKS VS. PATHOLOGICAL LESIONS

Our greatest glory is not in never failing, but
in rising every time we do fail.

Confucius

In many radiographs the shadows of bony structures, air sinuses, and foramina in bone are present in the areas that you would expect to find them. However, there are times when these shadows are projected onto the film in such a manner that one or more of them is superimposed over the root apex of a tooth. The resultant image closely resembles that of a pathological lesion and could be misinterpreted as such. No doubt countless numbers of teeth have been subjected to endodontic treatment or even extracted as a result of this misinterpretation.

There is a general rule to follow that will aid you toward a correct radiographic interpretation when a questionable area is observed. Always look for the periodontal ligament space and the lamina dura within the borders of the questionable shadow. If these two structures are present and normal in appearance, you can be sure that the shadow is not originating from a diseased tooth. (See Fig. 19–1A). A corollary to this would be that if these two structures are destroyed or altered in appearance, you can most assuredly conclude that the involved tooth is diseased and giving origin to the apical shadow in question. (See Fig. 19–1B).

If there is still some question in your mind, place another film in exactly the same position as before. Using the same vertical angulation as for the previous exposure, vary the horizontal angulation approximately 20 degrees either anteriorly or posteriorly. If the shadow still appears at the root apex in the same position as that seen on the original radiograph, it is probably representative of pathology arising from

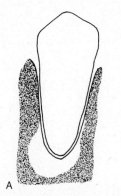 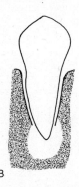

Figure 19–1 *A*, Questionable shadow at root apex has normal periodontal membrane space and lamina dura within its boundary. The shadow is not caused by a diseased tooth. *B*, Periodontal membrane space and lamina dura are discontinuous within the boundary of the questionable shadow. The involved tooth is diseased.

the involved tooth. However, if the shadow moves from its original position in relation to the tooth apex, it is probably a normal anatomic structure in the bone. Clinical examination of the tooth is most important, with emphasis placed on vitality tests.

The anatomical structures most likely to be involved in radiographic misinterpretation are as follows.

INCISIVE CANAL FORAMEN

As it usually appears on the radiograph, one has the impression that this foramen is located between the root tips of the maxillary central incisors. In actuality, the foramen opens on the midline of the palate at a position slightly below the apical level of the incisor teeth (Fig. 3–3A). Because of the vertical angle of x-ray projection for the maxillary central incisor exposure, the shadow of the foramen is located between the apices of the incisor teeth. This is especially true when using the bisection of the angle technique (Fig. 19–2). It takes only a slight shift in horizontal angulation from the midline to move the shadow over the apex of one of the central incisors (Fig. 19–3). Because of the radiolucent appearance of the foramen, one might easily get the impression that the tooth is pathologically involved.

MENTAL FORAMEN

The situation here is much the same as that described for the incisive canal foramen. Radiographically, the mental foramen is most frequently found between the apices of the mandibular bicuspids (Fig.

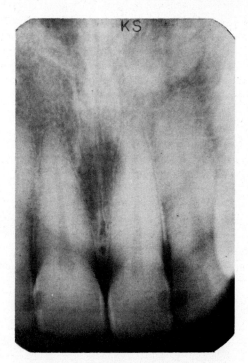

Figure 19-2 The shadow of the incisive canal foramen is most often seen between the apices of the central incisor teeth.

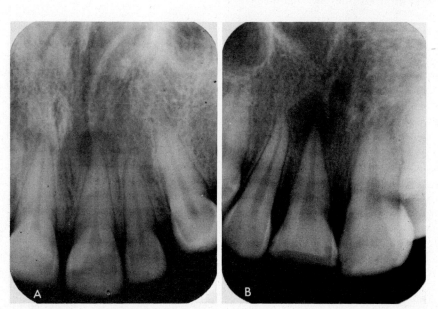

Figure 19-3 *A,* Owing to the off-angled direction of the horizontal angulation, the shadow of the incisive canal foramen is cast over the apex of the maxillary central incisor tooth, closely resembling the appearance of a diseased tooth. *B,* Radiolucent shadow at the apex of the right maxillary central incisor represents a diseased pulp. Note the discontinuity of the periodontal ligament space and the lamina dura over the apex of the tooth.

19–4A). There are many radiographs in which this foramen is superimposed over the root apex of either the first or second mandibular bicuspid. In actuality it is located on the labial surface of the mandible (Fig. 3–8A).

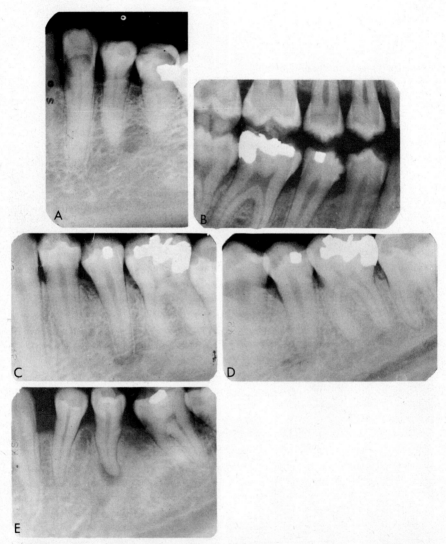

Figure 19–4   A, The shadow of the mental foramen is most often seen between the apices of the mandibular bicuspid teeth. B, Bite-wing radiograph does not exhibit any carious lesions of any significance. C, A periapical radiograph reveals a radiolucent area at the apex of the mandibular second bicuspid. Note the normal periodontal ligament space and the lamina dura. D, Supplemental periapical radiograph exposed with a 20-degree variation with the horizontal angulation. Note that the radiolucent area is no longer associated with the apex of the second bicuspid. E, Mandibular second bicuspid shows evidence of periapical pathology. Note the discontinuity of the periodontal ligament space and the lamina dura over the apex.

Let us observe a case history. The patient complained of moderate pain in the mandibular left second bicuspid, especially upon awakening in the morning. Clinically the oral tissues appeared to be in good health, although there were some areas of localized gingivitis. The second bicuspid in question and the first molar showed a mesial tilt. The mesial marginal ridge of the second bicuspid was well below the distal marginal ridge of the first bicuspid. At first glance the occlusion of these teeth with the maxillary teeth was basically good. There were no clinical caries.

On the bite-wing exposure there were no carious lesions of any significance (Fig. 19–4B). The mesial tilt of the second bicuspid was evident, with visible angular bone loss. On a routine periapical film (Fig. 19–4C), a radiolucent area was found at the apex of the second bicuspid. Under magnification the periodontal membrane and lamina dura were normal in appearance through the radiolucency. This observation ruled out the possibility of the radiolucency's being a pulp-derived pathosis from this tooth.

Of vital importance is that you remember that a very important radiolucent landmark is seen in this immediate area. It is the mental foramen. Because of the symptoms of the tooth, it was thought that an accurate pulp vitality test could not be obtained at this time. As a double check, a supplemental periapical radiograph was exposed with a variation of 20 degrees in the horizontal angulation (Fig. 19–4D). Notice that the radiolucent area is no longer associated with the apex of the second bicuspid. All apical structures appear normal and healthy in this radiograph—further proof that the area in question is the mental foramen. If the radiolucency was an abscess or granuloma, it would still appear radiolucent and attached to the apex, and the periodontal ligament space and the lamina dura would be obliterated within the radiolucency (Fig. 19–4E).

Pathology was ruled out, and upon reconsideration of the patient's complaint that the pain was felt upon awakening, it was determined that the patient was bruxating while sleeping. An occlusal adjustment was performed and there were no further symptoms.

MAXILLARY SINUS

When a patient presents a maxillary sinus of normal size or larger, you will often find that in radiographs of this area the roots of the molars and bicuspids appear to be projecting up into the sinus (Fig. 19–5A).

Actually the roots are positioned in alveolar bone and the hard palate, but owing to the angle of the x-ray beam projection, the roots and the sinus are superimposed one over the other. The shadow of the

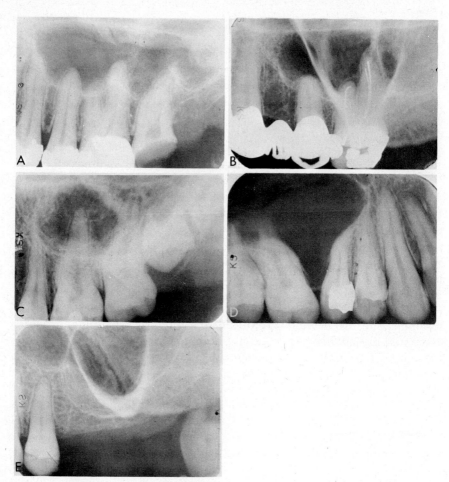

Figure 19–5 *A,* The roots of the teeth appear to be projecting into the sinus. *B,* Bone septa contrasting with sinus proper may simulate pathology. *C,* Configuration of bone within the maxillary sinus may simulate pathology. *D,* Expansion of sinus into alveolar bone. *E,* Expansion of sinus into alveolar bone. Note the radiolucent line, which represents a nutrient canal. The coronoid process is visible in the lower posterior corner of the radiograph.

sinus, being radiolucent and almost always containing bony septa, simulates the appearance of cyst formation when positioned over the apex of one or more roots. Adding to the problem are accessory compartments of the sinus and the malar bone shadows (Fig. 19–5*B* and *C*).

A radiograph often reveals an extra clue to the nature of the radiolucency. The normal maxillary sinus usually presents visible nutrient canals, which appear as darker bands or lines traversing within its boundaries. When these canals are observed, the radiolucent area is the sinus. Many radiographs of the maxillary molar region show expansion of the sinus into areas of missing teeth. This is most frequently seen when the first permanent molars were removed at an early age. The area of sinus expansion into the alveolar process surrounded by the radiopaque roots of the adjacent teeth may produce sharp contrasts between these structures that could possibly give rise to a misinterpretation. However, this is a normal process. (See Fig. 19–5D and E.)

SUBMAXILLARY GLAND FOSSA

This landmark appears as a broad radiolucent area below the root apices of the mandibular molars (Fig. 19–6). Being a depression in bone, more x-rays penetrate the area than penetrate the thicker surrounding bone. Unless the teeth are diseased, the lamina dura and periodontal ligament space surrounding the roots of each tooth are normal and intact. A questionable area of this size should always be checked to see if the appearance is bilateral. It is rare to find similar looking pathologic lesions bilaterally in opposing areas.

CORONOID PROCESS

This structure, when visible on a radiograph, is always seen in the maxillary third molar exposure. The patient has opened wide to facilitate film placement, which allows the coronoid process to rock forward to a position adjacent to the maxillary tuberosity. Consequently these two structures often appear superimposed over each other on the radiograph.

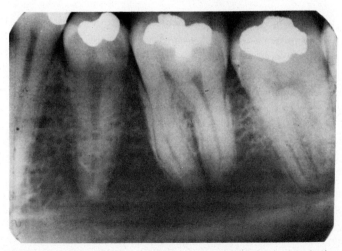

Figure 19–6   Broad radiolucent area below the mandibular molars is the submaxillary gland fossa.

Being mostly dense cortical bone, this process can resemble a root fragment. Knowledge that this structure does appear in this exposure and comparing densities between it and adjacent teeth enables you to make a correct interpretation. (See Fig. 19–7A and B.)

CEMENTOMA

The next entity in this series is not a case of misinterpreting a normal anatomical landmark as disease, but is a true pathological lesion. It is included in this series because in its beginning stages it resembles a periapical abscess or granuloma. It does not, however, require any

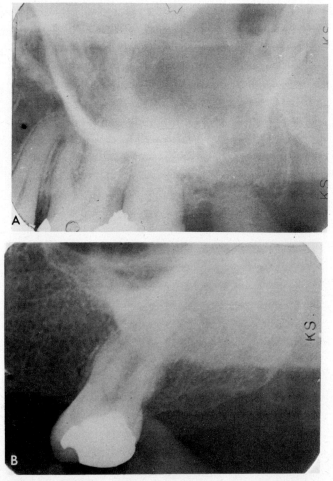

Figure 19–7 A, Maxillary molar radiograph with the coronoid process superimposed over the maxillary tuberosity. B, Coronoid process is seen superimposed over the distal surface of the maxillary molar.

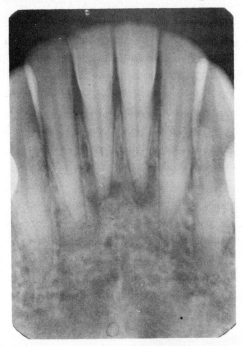

Figure 19-8   Mandibular central incisors are involved with a cementoma. The two central incisors show the early fibrotic stage (radiolucent). The right lateral incisor shows the later, healing stage in which the fibrotic tissue has been replaced with cementum.

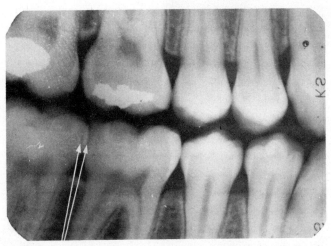

Figure 19-9   Radiolucent lines caused by overlapping enamel surfaces.

treatment. Though there are histologic changes, it is self-limiting by nature.

For some unknown reason, bone surrounding the root apex is replaced by fibrous tissue. The lesion appears radiolucent and may remain in this state for a protracted period of time or it may fill in with bone or cementum. We are interested only in the fibrotic or beginning stage, since this is the one that is almost always misinterpreted as an abscess or granuloma (Fig. 19–8).

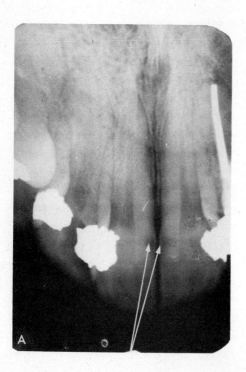

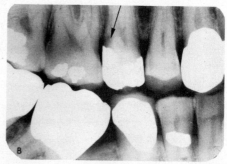

Figure 19–10 *A,* Radiolucent shadow represents cervical burnout. *B,* Cervical burnout under proximal restoration simulates recurrent caries.

Illustration continued on opposite page

By checking the vitality of the teeth, you can eliminate the possibility of a missed diagnosis. Teeth that are involved with a cementoma only are always vital. They nearly always occur in women in the 30- to 50-year-old age group. The mandibular anterior teeth are most frequently involved.

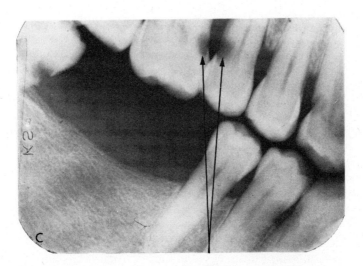

Cervical caries

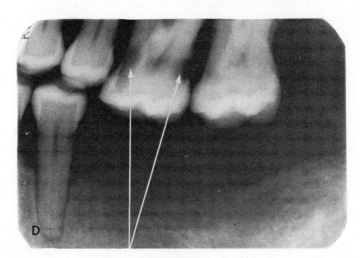

Cervical caries

Figure 19–10 *Continued.*   *C,* Cervical caries involving the cuspid, second bicuspid, and molars. Note destruction of the alveolar bone resulting from periodontal disease. *D,* Cervical caries involving the maxillary first molar. Note the break in the tooth surface and the expanding diffuse outline of the caries. Also note the extent of alveolar bone destruction.

Because of the vitality of the teeth, this lesion must not be misinterpreted as a foramen.

RADIOLUCENT AREAS OF TEETH

Though not considered major anatomical landmarks, the normal radiolucency of the cervical areas and interproximal contacts of the teeth can be misinterpreted as caries. The two conditions causing these questionable effects are interproximal overlap of enamel surfaces and cervical burnout.

There are many instances, especially on bite-wing radiographs, when two interproximal surfaces will overlap. This can be due to the natural overlap of misaligned teeth or to faulty horizontal angulation of the tube head. In either case, the overlapping projects an image of a dense radiopaque area. Immediately surrounding the overlapped enamel surfaces are faint radiolucent lines (Fig. 19–9). These lines are an optical illusion caused by the contrast between the normal appearing enamel and the area of dense overlapped enamel. Because of the contrast, the lines seem more lucent than they actually are. This is often spoken of as the "mach band" effect. Be alert to this so as not to interpret these radiolucent lines as incipient caries.

Cervical burnout is not an optical illusion necessarily, but the effect is often interpreted as cervical caries. Again, we have an area of lesser density interposed between two structures of greater density. Owing to the angle of x-ray projection, the resultant image is one of a radiolucent triangle at the cervical area of the tooth. This triangular area is the shadow of a portion of the tooth where the radiopaque enamel feathers out to a point at the junction of the root to where dense radiopaque cortical bone is seen. The structure and shape of the root in this area also allows for greater penetration of x-rays—hence, the radiolucent shadow (Fig. 19–10A). Be alert so as not to interpret this effect as cervical caries or as recurrent caries when seen under the proximal surface of a restoration (Fig. 19–10B).

Clinical exploration will usually resolve any question as to whether the area is carious or not. Also, if the periodontal structures are in a state of good health and the gingival attachment closely approximates the enamel, the area is almost always cervical burnout. Cemental caries rarely form under these healthy conditions.

Cemental caries, however, can appear in the same area of the tooth as cervical burnout. When they occur, you will note that the patient has a detached gingival margin and there is almost always some degree of alveolar crest destruction—in other words, advanced periodontal disease.

Cervical caries reveal an actual break in the tooth surface with a spreading diffuse outline (Fig. 19–10C and D). Again, probing the area clinically settles the question.

20

EIGHTY-FIVE PER CENT OF YOUR SUCCESS – YOUR PERSONALITY

All that a man achieves and all that he fails to achieve is the direct result of his own thoughts.

James Allen

It is the fondest wish of the author that this chapter, though not directly related to the mechanics of x-ray technique, will aid you in your endeavors to be outstanding in your chosen field. Because of the importance of the subject matter, many hours have been spent in trying to accentuate the most important points and yet keep the number of pages to a minimum. This is done to avoid overshadowing the main subject of the book.

Those of you who have been working in the dental field for a time know that there is much more to your work than the bare mechanics in performing certain procedures. You are a servant to the patients of your practice. You have been and will be meeting a variety of patients, each living in his or her own world. Much of your success will depend on how well you can adapt and communicate with each patient.

Before we progress any further, let me make one important point clear: YOU are a very vital part of the dental office with which you are associated. The way YOU adjust to the many different types of patients can literally make a good dental practice outstanding. YOU can also treat patients in such a manner that they may hesitate to ever return for further dental work. Just remember the earlier visits you have made to your own dentist and the manner in which you were treated by those in the office other than the dentist. What impression did you have of these auxiliary personnel? As you look back on these appointments, can you think of any constructive criticism you could offer to anyone in the office with regard to the way you were treated? Try to remember how much importance YOU placed on the manner in which YOU were personally treated.

This all leads up to the fact that if you are not already, you must now become adept in the subject of human relations. Many studies have proved beyond any doubt the truth of this statement. The Carnegie Institute of Technology made one such study in which records of 10,000 persons were analyzed. From all the data collected and studied, it was definitely determined that 15 per cent of the total success of these people was determined by their technical ability and skills on the job. The remaining 85 per cent was attributable to personality factors and the ability to communicate with people successfully.

The Bureau of Vocational Guidance at Harvard University made a study of thousands of men and women who had been fired. They found that for every three people who were fired from their jobs, two were released because of their inability to deal with people successfully.

You have put what seems like endless hours into studying and preparing for your career. To realize that this preparation will count a mere 15 per cent toward your success may come as quite a shock. However, the sooner you are aware of this, the better off you will be. By far the greatest portion of your success is going to depend upon your personality and your successful relationships with other people.

The author in no way professes to be an expert in human relations. Of the following points to be discussed you have probably heard many mentioned before. It is the purpose of this discussion to reemphasize the importance of each point and to indicate how to apply this knowledge in your work. If you will make each principle habitual with your total personality make-up and provide the best service possible to your employer and patients, your success should be more than assured.

THE MOST IMPORTANT WORD

Any discussion that involves the personality make-up of an individual must begin with a very basic aspect of that person. This basic aspect can be defined in one word—ATTITUDE. Your attitude, more than anything else, will determine the degree of your success or failure in life. We are talking not only about your success in your career but about life in general.

Webster defines attitude as "position or bearing as indicating action, feeling, or mood, hence the feeling or mood itself." From this definition we can see that spoken words are not necessary to convey one's attitude to another. People can sense your attitude by your posture and facial expression, and by the way you walk and behave. Your deepest inner feelings toward anything in your life will determine your attitude toward that thing.

For example, let's suppose you are faced with the task of learning a method for performing a new technique. If you approach the task with the idea that you can do it and that you will do it to the best of your ability, you have a "good attitude," and there is no question that the final outcome will yield outstanding results. Obviously the person with a poor attitude will not produce good results with any consistency. You can prove this to yourself. Just take a few moments to look back over some of the subjects you took in school. Generally the courses you enjoyed taking and in which you were most interested were those for which you received the best marks. You actually wanted to learn these subjects, and therefore they were the easiest for you. Being a good student, you probably received good marks in your other subjects as well, but I think you'll agree that you had to work a little harder in these courses. You'll always produce your finest results in those areas of work you like doing the most. It is easy to develop a good attitude toward your career if you enjoy the work. Your attitude will keep you moving forward when things don't seem to be going well.

Take a look at the people you know in the business and professional world. Notice that the more successful the person is, the better is his attitude toward his work. He is always asking himself how he can more effectively serve his patients, customers, or clients. He is very easy to talk with and can make you feel at ease instantly. He has a natural air about him that expresses confidence, poise, and sincerity in everything he does. Such people naturally move to top positions as if pulled by some magnetic force.

When you maintain a good positive attitude from day to day, you are assuring yourself a bright future. Why is this true? Because you will be following a law which is immutable: "As you sow, so shall you reap." Another way of stating the law is: "As you think, so shall you be." No matter how good your attitude is, it can always be better. Nothing in this world is being done in the very best way it can ever be done. There is always a better way that will replace the present one. You can use this fact to constantly improve yourself. You must also be aware that this law is working constantly. You are producing either good results (good attitude) or poor results (poor attitude). With a good attitude, one success is followed by another, each one a building block toward your ever-expanding accomplishments.

How you think determines exactly how you will act. When you answer the telephone, your "Good morning, this is Dr. Wonderful's office" will convey to the person on the other end of the line exactly how you feel about your place of service. You have said but seven words. However, the way you said them, the tone of your voice, and your enthusiasm tell the prospective patient, "I appreciate your calling this office; you are important and we want to serve you." Or your voice may imply just the opposite without your realizing it. If you ever have the opportunity to record your voice on a tape recorder, do so. You should find it quite revealing.

The process of improving one's attitude begins within the mind of the individual. Your ideas for improving your attitudes must be accepted mentally before they can ever be expressed physically.

To begin, you must first know your good points as well as the bad ones. Take a good long unbiased look at yourself. Above all, be honest. Do you like what you see? If not, why not? Make a list of your undesirable traits, and on the opposite side of the page list what you think you can do to correct these faults. Some may require more thought, and there may be more than one solution. If you feel it necessary, seek advice from a competent person. Be sure this person has YOUR INTEREST at heart and can give you genuine advice.

Make a plan for molding yourself into a better, more useful you. Then make sure you follow through with your plan. Decide on the person you would most like to be if you could change yourself instantly. Use your imagination. Picture yourself as having complete confidence and poise in all situations. See yourself performing your duties in a calm, cheerful manner. Keep this newly formed self-image constantly before you as you go about your daily routine. By doing this you will be constructing a good positive attitude, first toward yourself and then toward others as well. You will be sowing the seeds of a new and brighter attitude that will reap a new and brighter life for you. The great William James of Harvard University said, "The greatest discovery of my generation is that people can alter their lives by altering their attitudes of mind."

In your career you will be in contact with people who have widely varying mental and emotional make-ups. You will meet business executives, clerical personnel, professional people, teachers, students, and many others. Observe them and you will note that one of the most outstanding characteristics of a top-notch person is the way he or she treats other people. Regardless of the other person's station in life, give each the same courteous treatment consistently. Putting the other person's interest first is an absolute must for you when dealing with people. This is building a good attitude toward others in its truest sense.

DEVELOPING ENTHUSIASM

Another very important part of your total personality is absolutely necessary to develop if you wish to be effective in your contacts with others. Again, it is quite noticeable in people occupying the top echelons in their respective fields.

Did you ever hear one of your friends speak of an acquaintance as having a "vibrant personality" or an "overabundance of energy," or as just "glowing with life"? Do you know what trait your friend is describing? That's right . . . it is ENTHUSIASM!

Enthusiasm is from the Greek word *enthusiastes,* which is composed of two parts, *en,* which means in (or in the power of), and *theos,* which means god.* In other words, people who are enthusiastic are expressing the GOD POWER within them that manifests itself as a vibrant life, with energy to burn and the power to do anything they wish to do.

If you are lacking enthusiasm toward your work, you probably don't look forward to each day as you should. Before too long, this frame of mind will make you feel that you are in the proverbial rut. However, you must realize that it is not always the job or type of work you do that causes you to feel this way. In all probability it is your mental attitude toward your work that is the disturbing factor. It is this attitude that must be altered. This can be done by obtaining all the knowledge you can about your work. Challenge yourself to become an expert in whatever it is you are doing. Set goals for yourself and, once they are accomplished, keep setting new ones. These goals do not have to be earthshaking. Small personal goals will be enough to give you the feeling that you are progressing.

Setting goals gives you something to be enthusiastic about. But to really become an enthusiastic person you must begin by forcing yourself to act enthusiastically. Put life into your actions and your speech. Walk with a lively step and always check your posture, whether standing or sitting. Keep reminding yourself to act enthusiastically. As you pursue this course of action you will find that each day will bring about a change in you. The change may be ever so slight, but you will be building a new habit pattern. Before long you will no longer have to remind yourself to act in this new way, for your subconscious mind will take over your conscious actions and you will automatically react to everything with enthusiasm. Do you remember that when you were learning to drive you were very cautious and gave each move plenty of thought before performing it? Now you perform these movements without giving them a second thought. Developing enthusiasm works in the same manner.

The next time you are out with a group of people notice how many of them behave enthusiastically. Notice how many people in the dental field are genuinely enthusiastic. I don't think you will find too many. This is why it is so easy for you to succeed. With this in mind, make yourself into the person you know you can be. Live it up: Be ENTHUSIASTIC!

---

*Funk, W.: Word Origins and Their Romantic Stories. New York, Grosset & Dunlap, 1950.

FIRST IMPRESSIONS

Your good attitude and enthusiasm will surely influence others favorably, but of course the first impression is made by your appearance. Following are a few rules pertaining to grooming that should be followed when you are working in a dental office.

Most dentists require that you wear a uniform of some type. Make sure yours fits correctly and that it is always sparkling clean. A missing button or a slip that shows is sloppy. Stockings should always be worn, but whether or not they are white depends upon the wishes of your dentist. The type of shoes you wear is also up to your employer. If white ones are not required, select a pair of inconspicuous flats. You will be on your feet most of the day, and high heels would be very uncomfortable. If you wear street clothes rather than a uniform, let simplicity be the rule. Frilly blouses and dresses or extreme fashions would certainly be out of place. Simple jewelry is appropriate, but it should not be worn with your uniform.

Careful attention must be given to your personal cleanliness and grooming. You will be working in confined quarters in close proximity to the patient, so you must be sure you don't offend with unpleasant body odors. The use of heavy perfumes is not advisable either. Make-up should be used sparingly. Save the exotic eye make-up for an evening on the town. The same restraint should be shown when you arrange your hair-do. Wear it in a simple, easy-to-fix style when you are in the office. Your hands and fingernails should always be immaculately clean and well manicured. Patients pay particular attention to hands, since you will be handling the instruments that are placed in their mouths.

It's a good idea to scrutinize your appearance in a full-length mirror before leaving for work. Being happy with your outward appearance will add to your self-confidence. But if you are careless in this regard, it will be difficult to overcome the visual impression you make, even if your attitude is excellent and your enthusiasm boundless!

EFFECTIVE CONVERSATION

As we have learned, your attitude and enthusiasm can be expressed to others in many ways. However, the most obvious way in which we communicate with others is by conversation. If you will follow a few basic rules, I'm sure you will increase your effectiveness as a conversationalist, and at the same time you will become a very popular person with those you meet.

Do You Listen?   Have you ever tried to figure out why one person is more special to you than another? A very good reason is that he probably listens to you when you talk. That's all — he simply lends you an ear when you speak to him. When I say listen, I mean that he is attentive. He stops everything and anything he is doing to give you the special attention you deserve. When you leave his presence you feel that he is a very fine person. And yet all he did was to listen to you in a sympathetic way. If you carefully recall the moments you were together, I think you will find that the amount of talking you did was far in excess of the amount he did.

This is an extremely important lesson to learn. When conversing with a patient, treat him as though he were the most important person in the world. Take my word for it, to himself he *is* the most important person in the world. If you are preoccupied with something else, you must learn to stop whatever it is you are doing for the time being. Don't clean instruments or clear off the bracket table. It is an insult to the person to talk with him while you are trying to think about or do something else. If you find that you have been guilty of doing this, you have been indirectly telling the patient that what he has to say isn't important enough to demand your full attention. Don't for a moment think that patients are not aware of this. If, on the other hand, you follow through with this principle of undivided attention, you will soon acquire a reputation for being one of the wisest, most intelligent people around.

You have no doubt heard that you should sincerely compliment people as a means of getting them to think more favorably of you. This is true, but the point I would like to make here is that the most appreciated compliment is not necessarily a verbal compliment. What greater tribute can you pay to anyone than to give him your undivided attention? Whatever the other person is saying must be regarded as important, for if it weren't important to him, he wouldn't be saying it!

There are two ways to listen to someone. One is to listen with your ears, but the true listener listens with his eyes as well. If someone is talking to you, LOOK AT HIM. Don't let your eyes wander. Listen in an "eye-to-eye" manner, even if you must force yourself to do this. It will demonstrate your own confidence and poise. Also, check your posture. Don't lean or slouch, for this tends to indicate indifference. Stand or sit erect, or, if you must lean, lean toward the person speaking in order to accentuate your interest in what he is saying.

To further impress the person who is talking, ask him to repeat a statement now and then, or better still, ask questions pertaining to what he is telling you. This is proof that you are listening. You are also encouraging him to keep talking. How flattering can you get?

It is common knowledge that the majority of us would rather do the talking most of the time. Each of us has his own desires, opinions, and ideas that he would like to express. That is why it is so difficult to listen attentively without thinking ahead to what you are going to say. Being a good listener requires self-control and patience, but it is worth any effort you put forth to develop this quality in your personality.

The Verbal Compliment. The need for recognition and praise is probably the greatest need known to mankind. We have just stressed one way of truly complimenting another by attentive listening. However, a correctly used verbal compliment can be just as effective.

What you must avoid is insincere flattery. Don't say something nice to someone when both of you know the comment is partially or completely untrue. Most people will readily detect this as insincere. If this happens, you will have a hard time winning back that person's confidence in you. You must be sincere in your conversation with other people. Every patient who comes into the dental office deserves the same attention, regardless of how you may feel about him. It is very surprising how giving one sincere compliment at the proper time can change a person for the better and can change your own attitude toward him as well. Make your compliments specific. Don't compliment the person in general, but choose something about him or his appearance that is worth a favorable comment. If you are sincere in your efforts, you will find that everyone with whom you come in contact has at least one or two good points worthy of comment.

Many patients coming into the office will be reserved and quiet. Their conversation is limited to one- or two-word answers to your preliminary questions. Such reactions are probably due in part to the apprehension or anxiety they may feel because of the impending dental examination. In any case, a good method to bring such a patient out of his shell is to ask questions that cannot be answered with a "yes" or "no," such as "How did you get into this type of work?" or "How did you decide to go to that school?" What you are trying to do is to divert his mind from whatever is bothering him. Once this is accomplished, the problem usually reverses itself after an appointment or two. He will be so pleased with his newly discovered conversational ability that you might wish you had never got the conversation rolling in the first place!

The "ask a question" routine works especially well with children. Once the shy, apprehensive child knows he has a friend in these new and different surroundings he becomes a changed person. Also, children, like adults, appreciate sincere compliments.

Some patients may be easy to talk with one day and may tend to "clam up" the next. You may find this true with business executives who have pressing deadlines, with housewives who have problems on the home front, or even with a high school student who has just broken off with his best girl. You know that these people do not ordinarily act this way. Learn to sense their preoccupations. They certainly don't mean to be rude, but they do have problems that day and wish "to get the show on the road and get it over with." Take the hint and don't try to force a conversation. Make sure you do your part to keep things moving straight ahead. Tomorrow is another day in which you will find them their old selves again. You can be sure your efforts to go along with their moods are appreciated. Don't be offended or think that you may have precipitated the change from normal. After experiencing this situation a few times you will learn how to react. Working with a variety of people is an education in itself. It is a matter of developing a little empathy as well as sympathy.

A word of warning. Under no circumstance should you use gossip as a trigger for conversation. As far as you are concerned, make gossip taboo. Keep it forever out of the office. No matter how tempting the subject, avoid it. If you can't find something nice to say about someone, then don't say anything. If a patient involves you in such a conversation, try to change the subject. You will be greatly admired for this personality trait.

The "King's English."   As you enter a room you may be a lovely sight to behold. You may perform your duties to perfection. You may have developed the art of being a good listener. Your ability to give sincere compliments has won you many friends. But what next? What happens when it's your turn to talk? Do you speak in a warm, friendly, confident manner? Do you have a commanding knowledge of the English language? Your manner of speaking and the words you use greatly determine the amount of polish you will put on your personality. Anyone who has taken the time to develop good grammar and an ever-expanding vocabulary impresses those with whom he speaks. It has been shown that no matter what position a person holds, the one holding the position just above his on the ladder of success has just that much more knowledge of the correct use of words.

Again, as in anything else you wish to accomplish, effort is necessary to build your vocabulary beyond that which you use daily. Learning new words and their use is done by hearing them spoken or by reading them in a book or magazine. If at all possible, write the new word down on paper and, if time permits, the sentence in which it was used. Knowledge of how to use the new word, as well as its definition, is a must if you are going to use it effectively. You can build yourself a sizable list of words in a short period of time by this method. As your list grows you will notice how rapidly your confidence in yourself is growing. No longer have you any apprehensions about conversing with others. Certainly these other people will be aware of your poise and confidence.

One final word about your voice. Always speak in a warm, relaxed manner. A tense person develops a degree of shrillness when speaking, and this can be irritating to the patient or to anyone else listening. It is unavoidable in any job, and especially in a dental office, that there will be times when you are rushed and tensed. It is then that you must make a conscious effort to maintain control of your voice. No matter how extreme the circumstances, never allow yourself to speak to a patient except with a pleasant voice that expresses confidence, enthusiasm, and sincerity. And don't forget to speak with your eyes as well as your lips. As you look at the patient, let your eyes sparkle. It makes your voice twice as effective, and it is positive therapy to the patient.

SOMETHING TO THINK ABOUT

Did you ever stop to think who pays your salary? The dentist for whom you work? Yes, he hands you your paycheck. But who pays the dentist? The patient, of course. The patient is, in reality, your employer. Can you see why it is so important for you to treat each and every one as though he were the most important person in the world? As we mentioned earlier, each patient feels exactly that way, and he expects to be treated as such. You must fulfill this desire for first-class treatment. Not only does your success depend upon it, but tomorrow's work and income depend upon it as well. Try to do your share to make the patient want to return to your dental office for further treatment and to recommend your practice to other prospective patients. You can easily do this by the use of two simple phrases that are music to his ears—his name and "thank you."

In most instances you will be meeting the patient for the first time when you call him from the reception room. It is here that you apply a cardinal principle of personal communication. Always use the patient's name when you address him. In order to maintain the necessary formality of the office you should use the proper title (such as Miss, Mrs., Mr., Doctor, Reverend, etc.). Unless you are a very close friend, always use the last name. This maintains the patient's dignity. Be sure your spelling and pronunciation of the name is correct. If you're not sure of either, don't hesitate to ask. This flatters the person because you have made a special effort to get it right.

When the appointment is terminated, get the patient's coat for him and help him into it. Accentuate your courtesy. Take a few extra seconds to smile and say a sincere "thank you" followed by his name. Look into his eyes as you say it with enthusiasm. This makes it very personal, and he will leave the office feeling like a million. Again, communicating with your eyes as well as your voice not only makes friends for you but is a definite asset in building the practice.

PLEASING THE BOSS

As you read and study your way through these chapters you are learning how to become the person you have always wanted to be, both professionally and personally. You are developing your skills in all areas of dentistry as well as in patient contact. If you wish to keep moving ahead, don't forget this most important point—please the boss! Regardless of what you have accomplished in the way of skills, you will not succeed at your job unless you achieve this goal.

Let's understand one thing before going any further. By pleasing your employer, you do not demean yourself or lower your personal standards. Some people have a natural tendency to resent authority.

They feel that if one attains a certain level of performance, or exceeds it, success will automatically be assured. What they don't realize is that one person's opinion of successful accomplishment is not always in agreement with another's. The prime question is, what does your employer think of your "on-the-job" performance? You will not get a raise in salary, advancement, and so forth just because you think you deserve it. The person who pays your salary has to think so also. You have to please someone besides yourself. Whether you like this idea or not is unimportant. Those who do not accept this fact will not succeed. The better jobs and pay raises that might have been theirs will be passed on to someone else.

No employer is perfect, and some are more difficult to work for than others. Whenever you question your employer's attitude and behavior, remember that he is responsible for making his practice a success. There are times when stress is high. Do your part to restore order and smoothness to the day; your willingness to help him through these times will not go unnoticed.

If you find yourself in a difficult situation, first make sure that you are not causing the problem, then try your best to find a solution. When, in spite of your efforts, things don't work out, look for a position elsewhere. If you have been a good employee, most employers will be aware of this and will allow you to part on a satisfactory basis with a good recommendation.

THE EXCEPTIONAL DENTAL TECHNICIAN

When discussing practice administration with many dentists, the subject of office personnel seems to occupy much of the conversation. Although there is rarely any disappointment expressed about the ability or efficiency of anyone in the office, there is also a lack of genuinely favorable comments. Very few employers feel that any one of their employees is exceptional. Wouldn't you like your dentist to have glowing comments about the way you perform your duties?

Most dentists operate on a strict schedule that demands the utmost in efficiency from everyone concerned with the practice. When you are working for a dentist, you should do everything possible to increase your overall efficiency. Your work—your service to the doctor, patient, and other personnel in the office—should always be your first concern. Your own likes and desires must come second. This is true not only in dentistry but in any field of work. While performing your duties, make sure that you always put forth your best efforts.

Each person in the office generally has definite assigned duties. The correct and expeditious fulfillment of your own duties is the service rendered in return for the salary you earn. This is accepted as the routine procedure no matter what your job may be. If a person does not meet certain standards, there is always someone else waiting to step in and take over.

But what makes someone outstanding in a particular job? Exceptional employees are those who not only are pleased with their work but also have developed a sense of security and well-being about their jobs. What is their secret? *They do more than they are asked or expected to do.* Of course this is related to the subject of attitude. People who always do more than they are asked have an excellent attitude toward their work and toward life in general. This habit is the very thing that will separate you from the mass of mediocrity. It is also the surest way to attract favorable attention from the dentist. You will be giving more than is required of you, and this cannot go unrecognized. If it seems that this effort is not appreciated where you are, don't let that deter you. Keep on putting forth your best performance and you will be attracted elsewhere into a much better position. It never fails. This is also an excellent way to keep your position secure within the office. You might keep in mind that if you never do any more than you are paid to do, then you really don't have any grounds to ask for or to expect a raise in salary.

While making the effort to do extra work, do so cheerfully. Don't allow yourself the luxury of self-pity if you feel you are not appreciated. Feeling sorry for yourself will completely neutralize the good effects that result from doing more than you are expected to do.

IT'S UP TO YOU

This chapter has encompassed only a few of the different components that, when joined together, help to make up a highly complex unit defined as personality. You should grasp the importance of constantly striving to improve your personality, for it will enhance your ability to get along well with others. People are here to stay, and it is through these people that your many varied wishes will be granted. Therefore, understanding them and their reactions to certain situations is just as necessary as getting them to understand you.

You are a part of the great profession of dentistry and can justifiably be proud of yourself. The growth of dentistry depends to a large degree upon your ability to grow with it. You must give part of yourself to it before you can ever expect dentistry to contribute to your well-being, either financially or personally.

In some mysterious way we are all guided into the position and work best suited for us. Therefore you must have been given the necessary ingredients to perform your tasks successfully. You definitely have what it takes. Prove it to yourself and to everyone else. You can do it, you know—It's Up To YOU!

INDEX

Note: Page numbers in *italics* refer to illustrations.

Abscesses, periapical, 213–216, *215*
Acetic acid, in fixing solution, 37
Alveolar bone, 41, 42, *42*
Alveolar crest, 41, *41*
Ammonia thiosulfate, in fixing solution, 37
Anatomical landmarks, 40–53. See also
    Mandibular arch and *Maxillary arch.*
  of mandibular arch, 49–53, *47–52*
  of maxillary arch, 42–49, *43–46*
  vs. pathological lesions, 227–238
Angström unit, 2
Angulations, horizontal, in exposing
  teeth, *59*
Anode, of x-ray tube, 21, *22, 23*
Arch(es). See *Mandibular arch* and
  Maxillary arch.
Arch morphology, abnormal, and bisection
  of angle technique, 116–122
  normal, and bisection of angle technique,
    122–129
Articular eminence, 180, *181, 182*
Atom(s), 4
  hydrogen, diagram of, *5*
  ionization of, 5, *5*
Automatic film processor, 37

Background radiation, 11
Bending, excessive, of x-ray film, 193, *195*
Bicuspids, anatomical landmarks near, in
    mandibular arch, *49,* 51–52
  in maxillary arch, *45,* 45–47
  apical abscess of, *215*
  bite-wing exposure of, 89–90, *90–92*
  periapical films of, 68, *72*
  in mandibular arch, 80, *82*
Bisection of angle technique, 54–62
  abnormal arch morphology and, 116–122
  equilateral triangle in, 54–57, *55, 56*
  in edentulous patients, 167, *168,*
    169–170
  paralleling technique vs., 96
    radiographs with, *109*

Bisection of angle technique (*Continued*)
  placement of film and tube head in,
    57–59, *57–59*
  problems with, 116–129
  review of basic principles for, 112–114
  taking of radiograph with, 59–61
  with narrow mandibular arch, 119–122
    bicuspid exposure, 122
    cuspid exposure, 121, *122*
    incisor exposure, 120–121
    molar exposure, 122
  with narrow "V"-shaped maxillary arch,
    116–119
    bicuspid exposure, 118, *118*
    bite-wing exposure, 119, *119, 120*
    cuspid exposure, 117, *118*
    incisor exposure, 117, *117*
    molar exposure, 119
  with variants of normal arches, 124–129
Bite-block film holder, 71, 76
  in mandibular arch, *86,* 87
  in maxillary arch, 75
Bite-wing exposures, *38,* 88–95
  anterior, 91, 93–95, *94*
  film for, 28, *29*
    sizes of, 29
  in children, 156–157, *157,* 163, *165*
  of bicuspids, 89–90, *90–92*
  of ectopically positioned teeth, 125, *126*
  of molars, 91, *92, 93*
  position of patient, film, and cone tip in,
    94, 95
Bite-wing tab, stabilization of, 93
Black film, 199, *200*
Blank film, 199
Bone, cancellous, 41, *41*
Bone sclerosis, 216, *218–219,* 220–221
Burnout, cervical, *236,* 238

Cancellous bone, 41, *41*
Caries, cervical, *237,* 238
  x-ray films and, 211, *212, 214*